THE ANTI-INFLAMMATORY LIFESTYLE: A COMPREHENSIVE GUIDE TO REDUCING INFLAMMATION AND OPTIMIZING HEALTH

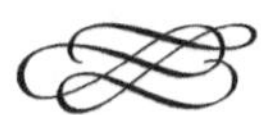

ALICE JENNER

UNDERSTANDING INFLAMMATION

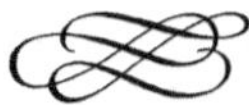

$\mathcal{I}$nflammation is a natural and essential process in the human body, playing a crucial role in healing and protecting us from harmful substances. However, when inflammation becomes chronic, it can lead to various health problems and diseases. In this chapter, we will delve into the concept of inflammation, differentiate between acute and chronic inflammation, explore the causes of chronic inflammation, and discuss the symptoms and health risks associated with prolonged inflammatory responses.

What is inflammation? Inflammation is the body's defense mechanism against injury, infection, or irritation. It is a complex biological response involving the immune system, blood vessels, and various molecular mediators. The primary purpose of inflammation is to eliminate the initial cause of cell injury, remove damaged cells and tissues, and initiate the healing process.

When the body detects a threat, such as a cut, sprain, or invasion by harmful microorganisms, the immune system is activated. White blood cells, particularly neutrophils and macrophages, are recruited to the affected area. These cells release chemical mediators called cytokines and chemokines, which cause blood vessels to dilate and become more permeable. This increased blood flow and permeability allows more immune cells and fluid to reach the site of injury or infection, causing the characteristic signs of inflammation: redness, swelling, heat, pain, and sometimes loss of function.

Acute vs. chronic inflammation Inflammation can be classified into two main types: acute and chronic. Acute inflammation is a short-term response that typically lasts a few days to a few weeks. It is a normal and beneficial process that helps the body heal and fight off infections. Examples of acute inflammation include:

1 A sprained ankle that becomes swollen and painful

2 A cut that becomes red and tender

3 A sore throat caused by a bacterial or viral infection

In these cases, the inflammatory response is triggered, the immune system works to resolve the issue, and the inflammation subsides once the healing process is complete.

On the other hand, chronic inflammation is a prolonged inflammatory response that can last for several months or even years. In this case, the body's immune system remains activated even when there is no apparent threat or injury. Chronic inflammation can be caused by various factors, such as an untreated infection, an autoimmune disorder, or long-term exposure to irritants. Some examples of conditions associated with chronic inflammation include:

1 Rheumatoid arthritis

2 Asthma

3 Inflammatory bowel disease (IBD)

4 Psoriasis

5 Chronic sinusitis

Chronic inflammation can lead to tissue damage, pain, and the development of various diseases, which we will discuss later in this chapter.

Causes of chronic inflammation Chronic inflammation can be caused by a variety of factors, both internal and external. Some of the most common causes include:

1 Untreated acute inflammation: When an acute inflammatory response is not resolved properly, it can progress into chronic inflam-

mation. This may occur due to an untreated infection or a foreign body that remains in the tissue.

2 Autoimmune disorders: In autoimmune diseases, the immune system mistakenly attacks the body's own tissues, leading to chronic inflammation. Examples include rheumatoid arthritis, lupus, and multiple sclerosis.

3 Chronic infections: Persistent infections, such as those caused by bacteria, viruses, or parasites, can trigger a prolonged inflammatory response. Examples include tuberculosis, hepatitis C, and Helicobacter pylori infection.

4 Long-term exposure to irritants: Repeated exposure to environmental toxins, pollutants, or chemicals can cause chronic inflammation. For example, long-term exposure to air pollution or industrial chemicals may lead to chronic respiratory inflammation.

5 Obesity: Excess body fat, particularly visceral fat around the abdominal organs, can trigger the release of pro-inflammatory chemicals, leading to chronic low-grade inflammation throughout the body.

6 Unhealthy dietary habits: A diet high in refined sugars, processed foods, and unhealthy fats (such as trans fats) can promote inflammation in the body. These foods can disrupt the balance of gut bacteria and increase the production of pro-inflammatory compounds.

7 Sedentary lifestyle: Lack of regular physical activity can contribute to chronic inflammation. Exercise has been shown to have anti-inflammatory effects by reducing body fat, improving insulin sensitivity, and promoting the release of anti-inflammatory cytokines.

8 Chronic stress: Prolonged psychological stress can lead to the overproduction of cortisol, a stress hormone that can promote inflammation when chronically elevated.

9 Aging: As we age, our immune system becomes less efficient and more prone to chronic low-grade inflammation, a condition known as "inflammaging."

Understanding the various causes of chronic inflammation can help individuals make lifestyle changes to reduce their risk of developing inflammation-related health problems.

Symptoms and health risks associated with chronic inflammation Chronic inflammation can manifest in various ways and affect multiple organ systems. Some common symptoms of chronic inflammation include:

1 Persistent fatigue

2 Joint pain and stiffness

3 Muscle aches

4 Headaches

5 Skin rashes or lesions

6 Gastrointestinal issues (e.g., bloating, diarrhea, or constipation)

7 Unexplained weight gain or weight loss

8 Frequent infections

9 Depression or mood disorders

It is essential to recognize that these symptoms can be nonspecific and may be associated with other health conditions. However, if you experience persistent symptoms that do not resolve on their own, it is crucial to consult a healthcare professional for proper evaluation and diagnosis.

Chronic inflammation has been linked to the development and progression of various diseases, including:

1 Cardiovascular disease: Chronic inflammation can damage blood vessels and contribute to the formation of atherosclerotic plaques, increasing the risk of heart attack and stroke.

2 Type 2 diabetes: Inflammation can lead to insulin resistance, a key factor in the development of type 2 diabetes. In turn, high blood sugar levels can further exacerbate inflammation, creating a vicious cycle.

3 Cancer: Chronic inflammation has been associated with an increased risk of certain cancers, such as colorectal, lung, and liver cancer. Inflammatory compounds can promote cell proliferation, survival, and migration, contributing to tumor growth and metastasis.

4 Neurodegenerative diseases: Inflammation in the brain has been linked to the development and progression of neurodegenerative diseases, such as Alzheimer's and Parkinson's.

5 Respiratory diseases: Chronic inflammation in the airways can

contribute to the development and exacerbation of respiratory conditions, such as asthma and chronic obstructive pulmonary disease (COPD).

6 Autoimmune disorders: As mentioned earlier, autoimmune diseases are characterized by chronic inflammation resulting from the immune system attacking the body's own tissues.

7 Chronic kidney disease: Inflammation can damage the kidneys and contribute to the progression of chronic kidney disease.

Understanding the health risks associated with chronic inflammation emphasizes the importance of addressing and managing this condition to maintain overall well-being and prevent the development of serious diseases.

In conclusion, inflammation is a complex biological response that plays a crucial role in protecting the body from harm. While acute inflammation is a normal and beneficial process, chronic inflammation can lead to various health problems and diseases. By understanding the causes and symptoms of chronic inflammation, individuals can take steps to reduce their risk factors and adopt lifestyle changes that promote an anti-inflammatory state. In the following chapters, we will explore the role of diet in inflammation and discuss how an anti-inflammatory diet can help manage and prevent chronic inflammation, ultimately supporting overall health and well-being.

INTRODUCTION TO THE ANTI-INFLAMMATORY DIET

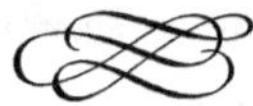

In the previous chapter, we discussed the concept of inflammation, the differences between acute and chronic inflammation, and the various health risks associated with prolonged inflammatory responses. As we have seen, chronic inflammation can contribute to the development and progression of numerous diseases, including cardiovascular disease, type 2 diabetes, cancer, and autoimmune disorders. Given the significant impact of inflammation on our health, it is crucial to explore strategies that can help manage and reduce chronic inflammation. One such approach is adopting an anti-inflammatory diet.

What is an anti-inflammatory diet? An anti-inflammatory diet is a way of eating that focuses on consuming foods that have been shown to reduce inflammation in the body while limiting or avoiding foods that can promote inflammatory responses. This dietary approach emphasizes whole, minimally processed foods that are rich in nutrients, antioxidants, and other beneficial compounds.

The anti-inflammatory diet is not a strict, one-size-fits-all eating plan but rather a set of guidelines that can be adapted to individual needs and preferences. The core principles of an anti-inflammatory diet include:

1 Eating a variety of fruits and vegetables: These foods are packed with vitamins, minerals, fiber, and phytochemicals that have anti-inflammatory properties. Aim to consume a rainbow of colorful produce to ensure you're getting a wide range of nutrients.

2 Choosing whole grains over refined grains: Whole grains, such as brown rice, quinoa, and whole wheat, contain more fiber and nutrients than their refined counterparts. Fiber helps maintain a healthy gut microbiome, which is essential for regulating inflammation.

3 Incorporating healthy fats: Omega-3 fatty acids, found in fatty fish, nuts, and seeds, have potent anti-inflammatory effects. Monounsaturated fats, found in olive oil and avocados, are also beneficial for reducing inflammation.

4 Selecting lean proteins: Lean proteins, such as fish, poultry, and plant-based sources (e.g., legumes and tofu), are preferred over red and processed meats, which have been linked to increased inflammation.

5 Limiting processed foods, refined sugars, and unhealthy fats: These foods can disrupt the balance of gut bacteria and promote inflammation throughout the body.

6 Using herbs and spices: Many herbs and spices, such as ginger, turmeric, garlic, and rosemary, have anti-inflammatory compounds that can add flavor to meals while providing health benefits.

By following these guidelines, an anti-inflammatory diet aims to provide the body with the nutrients it needs to maintain a healthy immune response and reduce chronic inflammation.

Benefits of an anti-inflammatory diet Adopting an anti-inflammatory diet can offer numerous health benefits, both in terms of managing existing inflammatory conditions and preventing the development of chronic diseases. Some of the key benefits include:

1 Reduced inflammation: By consuming foods that have anti-inflammatory properties and limiting those that promote inflammation, an anti-inflammatory diet can help reduce overall inflammation in the body.

2 Improved gut health: The high fiber content and beneficial

compounds found in whole foods can support the growth of healthy gut bacteria, which play a crucial role in regulating inflammation.

3 Better weight management: Anti-inflammatory foods tend to be nutrient-dense and filling, which can help with maintaining a healthy weight. Excess body fat, particularly visceral fat, can contribute to chronic inflammation.

4 Enhanced heart health: The anti-inflammatory diet emphasizes foods that are known to support cardiovascular health, such as fruits, vegetables, whole grains, and healthy fats. These foods can help lower blood pressure, improve cholesterol levels, and reduce the risk of heart disease.

5 Reduced risk of chronic diseases: By managing inflammation, an anti-inflammatory diet can help lower the risk of developing chronic diseases such as type 2 diabetes, certain cancers, and autoimmune disorders.

6 Improved symptom management: For individuals with existing inflammatory conditions, such as rheumatoid arthritis or inflammatory bowel disease, following an anti-inflammatory diet can help alleviate symptoms and improve overall quality of life.

7 Increased energy levels: Consuming nutrient-rich foods and reducing inflammation can lead to improved energy levels and reduced fatigue.

8 Better mental health: Inflammation has been linked to various mental health disorders, such as depression and anxiety. An anti-inflammatory diet may help support brain health and improve mood.

It's important to note that while an anti-inflammatory diet can offer significant health benefits, it should be used as part of a comprehensive approach to health and well-being. Regular physical activity, stress management, and adequate sleep are also essential for managing inflammation and promoting overall health.

How the diet works to reduce inflammation The anti-inflammatory diet works by targeting several key pathways and mechanisms involved in the inflammatory response. Here's a closer look at how the various components of the diet contribute to reducing inflammation:

1 Antioxidants: Fruits, vegetables, and whole grains are rich in antioxidants, such as vitamins C and E, beta-carotene, and polyphenols. These compounds help neutralize harmful free radicals that can damage cells and promote inflammation. Antioxidants also support the body's natural defenses against oxidative stress, which is a key driver of chronic inflammation.

2 Omega-3 fatty acids: Omega-3s, particularly EPA and DHA found in fatty fish, have potent anti-inflammatory effects. They work by reducing the production of pro-inflammatory compounds, such as cytokines and eicosanoids, and promoting the synthesis of anti-inflammatory mediators, such as resolvins and protectins.

3 Fiber: Dietary fiber, found in fruits, vegetables, whole grains, and legumes, supports the growth of beneficial gut bacteria. These bacteria produce short-chain fatty acids (SCFAs), such as butyrate, which have anti-inflammatory effects in the gut and throughout the body. Fiber also helps maintain the integrity of the gut lining, preventing the translocation of harmful bacteria and toxins that can trigger systemic inflammation.

4 Plant-based proteins: Legumes, nuts, and seeds are good sources of plant-based proteins that are also rich in anti-inflammatory compounds, such as fiber, polyphenols, and healthy fats. These proteins can help reduce inflammation by improving insulin sensitivity and promoting the production of anti-inflammatory cytokines.

5 Herbs and spices: Many herbs and spices contain potent anti-inflammatory compounds. For example, curcumin, the active ingredient in turmeric, has been shown to inhibit several inflammatory pathways and reduce markers of inflammation in the body. Ginger, garlic, and rosemary also have anti-inflammatory properties that can help modulate the immune response.

6 Limiting pro-inflammatory foods: By reducing the consumption of processed foods, refined sugars, and unhealthy fats, an anti-inflammatory diet helps minimize the intake of compounds that can promote inflammation. These foods can disrupt the balance of gut bacteria, increase oxidative stress, and activate pro-inflammatory signaling pathways.

The anti-inflammatory diet works by providing the body with a wide range of nutrients and bioactive compounds that work synergistically to modulate the immune response and reduce inflammation. By consistently following this dietary pattern, individuals can create a more balanced and resilient internal environment that is less prone to chronic inflammation and its associated health risks.

Success stories and testimonials While scientific evidence strongly supports the benefits of an anti-inflammatory diet, it is also helpful to consider real-life success stories and testimonials from individuals who have experienced the positive effects of this dietary approach firsthand. Here are a few examples:

1 Sarah, a 45-year-old woman with rheumatoid arthritis, had been struggling with joint pain and stiffness for years. After adopting an anti-inflammatory diet, she noticed a significant reduction in her symptoms within a few weeks. She reported increased energy levels, better mobility, and an overall improvement in her quality of life.

"I was skeptical at first, but I decided to give the anti-inflammatory diet a try. I was amazed at how quickly I started to feel better. My joint pain and stiffness decreased, and I had more energy throughout the day. I feel like I have my life back, and I'm so grateful for this dietary approach." - Sarah

2 John, a 55-year-old man with a family history of heart disease, decided to adopt an anti-inflammatory diet as a proactive measure to improve his cardiovascular health. After six months of following the diet, his blood pressure and cholesterol levels had improved significantly, and he had lost some excess weight.

"I knew I needed to make some changes to protect my heart health, and the anti-inflammatory diet seemed like a good place to start. I was pleasantly surprised by how much I enjoyed the foods and how satisfying the meals were. Seeing the improvements in my blood work and weight was a huge motivation to stick with the diet long-term." - John

3 Emily, a 32-year-old woman with inflammatory bowel disease, found that incorporating more anti-inflammatory foods into her diet helped manage her symptoms and reduce flare-ups. She reported less

abdominal pain, improved digestion, and a greater sense of control over her condition.

"Living with IBD can be challenging, but the anti-inflammatory diet has been a game-changer for me. By focusing on whole, nutrient-dense foods and limiting triggers, I've been able to better manage my symptoms and feel more in control of my health. It's not always easy, but the benefits are worth it." - Emily

4 Michael, a 28-year-old man who struggled with chronic fatigue and brain fog, decided to try an anti-inflammatory diet to see if it would improve his cognitive function and energy levels. After a few months, he reported clearer thinking, improved memory, and a significant boost in his overall well-being.

"I had been dealing with fatigue and brain fog for so long that I had almost accepted it as my new normal. The anti-inflammatory diet was a revelation for me. As I started to fuel my body with nutritious, anti-inflammatory foods, I noticed a marked improvement in my mental clarity and energy levels. I feel like I'm finally able to show up as my best self, both personally and professionally." - Michael

These success stories highlight the transformative potential of an anti-inflammatory diet for individuals with a wide range of health concerns. While individual results may vary, these testimonials demonstrate that making dietary changes can have a profound impact on overall health and well-being.

It's important to remember that adopting an anti-inflammatory diet is not a quick fix but rather a long-term commitment to nourishing your body with whole, nutrient-dense foods. It may take time to experience the full benefits, and there may be challenges along the way. However, with persistence, support, and a willingness to make sustainable lifestyle changes, many people find that an anti-inflammatory diet can be a powerful tool for improving their health and quality of life.

In the following chapters, we will delve deeper into the practical aspects of implementing an anti-inflammatory diet, including which foods to embrace, which foods to avoid, and strategies for meal planning and preparation. By understanding the science behind the diet and learning how to apply its principles in your daily life, you can take an active role in reducing inflammation and promoting optimal health.

INFLAMMATORY FOODS TO AVOID

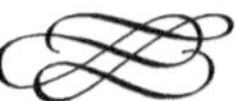

$\mathcal{I}$n the previous chapter, we introduced the concept of an anti-inflammatory diet and discussed its numerous bene-fits for managing chronic inflammation and promoting overall health. To fully embrace an anti-inflammatory lifestyle, it is essential to understand which foods can trigger or exacerbate inflammatory responses in the body. In this chapter, we will explore the main categories of inflammatory foods to avoid, including processed foods and refined sugars, saturated and trans fats, gluten and dairy sensitivities, high-glycemic foods, and food additives and preservatives.

Processed foods and refined sugars Processed foods and refined sugars are among the most significant contributors to chronic inflammation. These foods are often high in calories but low in essential nutrients, leading to weight gain and metabolic disturbances that can fuel inflammation.

Processed foods are typically manufactured using a combination of refined grains, added sugars, unhealthy fats, and artificial ingredients. Examples include packaged snacks, sugary cereals, candy, and soda. These foods are often stripped of their natural fiber, vitamins, and minerals, making them quickly digestible and more likely to cause rapid spikes in blood sugar levels. Over time, this can lead to insulin resistance, a key driver of inflammation and a precursor to type 2 diabetes.

Refined sugars, such as high fructose corn syrup and white sugar, are particularly problematic. When consumed in excess, these sugars can promote the formation of advanced glycation end products (AGEs), which are harmful compounds that can damage proteins and stimulate inflammation. Additionally, high sugar intake can disrupt the balance of gut bacteria, leading to a condition called dysbiosis, which has been linked to increased intestinal permeability (leaky gut) and systemic inflammation.

To minimize the inflammatory effects of processed foods and refined sugars, focus on consuming whole, minimally processed foods that are naturally rich in fiber, vitamins, and minerals. Choose fresh fruits and vegetables, whole grains, and lean proteins over packaged snacks and sugary treats. When reading food labels, be mindful of added sugars, which can appear under various names, such as sucrose, dextrose, and maltose.

Saturated and trans fats Saturated and trans fats are another group of inflammatory foods to avoid. While some saturated fats, such as those found in coconut oil and grass-fed beef, can be consumed in moderation, excessive intake of saturated fats has been linked to increased inflammation and cardiovascular disease risk.

Saturated fats are primarily found in animal-based foods, such as fatty cuts of meat, full-fat dairy products, and tropical oils (e.g., palm and coconut oil). When consumed in excess, saturated fats can increase levels of low-density lipoprotein (LDL) cholesterol, also known as "bad" cholesterol. High LDL levels can contribute to the formation of arterial plaques, which can trigger inflammatory responses and increase the risk of heart disease and stroke.

Trans fats, on the other hand, are considered the most harmful type of dietary fat. These fats are created through a process called hydrogenation, which turns liquid vegetable oils into solid fats at room temperature. Trans fats are commonly found in processed foods, such as packaged snacks, baked goods, and fried foods. Like saturated fats, trans fats can raise LDL cholesterol levels, but they also lower levels of high-density lipoprotein (HDL) cholesterol, or "good" cholesterol. This combination of effects can significantly increase inflammation and cardiovascular disease risk.

To minimize the inflammatory impact of saturated and trans fats, focus on consuming healthy, unsaturated fats from sources like olive oil, avocados, nuts, and fatty fish. These foods are rich in anti-inflammatory compounds, such as omega-3 fatty acids and monounsaturated fats, which can help reduce inflammation and support heart health.

Gluten and dairy sensitivities Gluten and dairy are two common food sensitivities that can trigger inflammatory responses in some individuals. While not everyone is sensitive to these foods, it is essential to be aware of their potential inflammatory effects and to pay attention to how your body responds to them.

Gluten is a protein found in wheat, barley, and rye. In people with celiac disease, an autoimmune disorder, consuming gluten triggers an immune response that damages the lining of the small intestine, leading to chronic inflammation and nutrient malabsorption. Even in individuals without celiac disease, gluten sensitivity or intolerance can cause digestive discomfort, headaches, fatigue, and other inflammatory symptoms.

Dairy products, such as milk, cheese, and yogurt, can also be problematic for some people. Lactose intolerance, which occurs when the body lacks the enzyme needed to digest the sugar in milk, can cause digestive issues and inflammation. Additionally, some individuals may be sensitive to the proteins in dairy, such as casein and whey, which can trigger inflammatory responses and exacerbate conditions like acne, eczema, and asthma.

If you suspect that gluten or dairy may be contributing to your inflammation, try eliminating these foods from your diet for a few weeks and observe any changes in your symptoms. You can then reintroduce them one at a time to assess your tolerance. If you find that gluten or dairy consistently triggers inflammatory symptoms, it may be best to avoid these foods and focus on nutrient-dense, anti-inflam matory alternatives, such as gluten-free grains (e.g., quinoa, rice, and oats) and plant-based milk and cheese.

High-glycemic foods High-glycemic foods are those that cause rapid spikes in blood sugar levels after consumption. These foods are quickly digested and absorbed, leading to a swift increase in glucose in the bloodstream. Over time, consistently consuming high-glycemic foods can contribute to insulin resistance, chronic inflammation, and an increased risk of type 2 diabetes and cardiovascular disease.

Examples of high-glycemic foods include:

1 White bread, pasta, and rice

2 Sugary breakfast cereals

3 Potatoes (especially mashed or french fries)

4 Sugary drinks, such as soda and fruit juices

5 Candy and desserts

When blood sugar levels rise quickly, the body releases insulin to help shuttle glucose into the cells. However, when this process occurs frequently due to a high-glycemic diet, the cells can become less responsive to insulin, leading to insulin resistance. This condition is characterized by persistently elevated blood sugar levels, which can fuel inflammation and oxidative stress throughout the body.

To minimize the inflammatory impact of high-glycemic foods, focus on consuming low-glycemic alternatives that are rich in fiber, protein, and healthy fats. These nutrients help slow down digestion and promote a more gradual release of glucose into the bloodstream. Examples of low-glycemic foods include:

1 Non-starchy vegetables (e.g., leafy greens, broccoli, and cauliflower)

2 Whole fruits (e.g., berries, apples, and pears)

3 Whole grains (e.g., quinoa, brown rice, and oats)

4 Legumes (e.g., lentils, chickpeas, and black beans)

5 Nuts and seeds

By replacing high-glycemic foods with these nutrient-dense, low-glycemic options, you can help regulate blood sugar levels, reduce inflammation, and support overall health.

Food additives and preservatives Food additives and preservatives are commonly used in processed foods to enhance flavor, texture, and shelf life. While some additives are considered safe, others have been linked to inflammatory responses and adverse health effects.

One group of food additives that has received significant attention in recent years is emulsifiers. These compounds, which include carboxymethylcellulose and polysorbate 80, are used to improve the texture and consistency of processed foods, such as ice cream, salad dressings, and baked goods. Studies have shown that emulsifiers can disrupt the gut microbiome, leading to increased intestinal permeability and inflammation. In animal studies, emulsifiers have been linked to the development of metabolic disorders, such as obesity and insulin resistance.

Another class of additives that can trigger inflammation is artificial sweeteners. While these compounds are often promoted as low-calorie alternatives to sugar, some studies suggest that they may disrupt the balance of gut bacteria and lead to glucose intolerance and inflammation. Common artificial sweeteners include aspartame, sucralose, and saccharin.

Preservatives, such as sodium benzoate and potassium sorbate, are added to foods to prevent spoilage and extend shelf life. While these compounds are generally considered safe, some individuals may be sensitive to them and experience inflammatory symptoms, such as headaches, skin irritation, and digestive issues.

To minimize your exposure to potentially inflammatory food additives and preservatives, focus on consuming whole, minimally processed foods that are free from artificial ingredients. When purchasing packaged foods, read labels carefully and choose products with short, recognizable ingredient lists. Additionally, consider preparing more meals at home using fresh, whole ingredients, as this allows you to control the quality and content of your food.

Conclusion In this chapter, we have explored the main categories of inflammatory foods to avoid, including processed foods and refined sugars, saturated and trans fats, gluten and dairy sensitivities, high-glycemic foods, and food additives and preservatives. By understanding the potential inflammatory effects of these foods and learning to identify them in your diet, you can take important steps toward reducing chronic inflammation and promoting optimal health.

It is important to remember that everyone's body is unique, and what triggers inflammation in one person may not have the same effect on another. Pay attention to how your body responds to different foods, and be willing to make adjustments as needed. If you have a pre-existing health condition or are considering making significant changes to your diet, it is always best to consult with a healthcare professional or registered dietitian for personalized guidance.

Adopting an anti-inflammatory diet is a journey that requires patience, commitment, and a willingness to experiment with new foods and flavors. In the coming chapters, we will explore the nutrient-dense, anti-inflammatory foods that can help nourish your body and support optimal health. By focusing on these health-promoting foods and minimizing your intake of inflammatory triggers, you can take a proactive approach to managing inflammation and enhancing your overall well-being.

ANTI-INFLAMMATORY FOODS TO EMBRACE

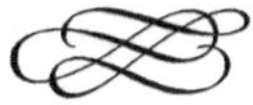

In the previous chapter, we discussed the various inflammatory foods to avoid in order to reduce chronic inflammation and promote optimal health. While minimizing your intake of these triggering foods is crucial, it is equally important to focus on incorporating nutrient-dense, anti-inflammatory foods into your diet. In this chapter, we will explore the key categories of anti-inflammatory foods to embrace, including fruits and vegetables, whole grains, healthy fats, lean proteins, herbs and spices, and fermented foods and probiotics.

Fruits and vegetables Fruits and vegetables are the cornerstone of an anti-inflammatory diet. These plant-based foods are rich in vitamins, minerals, antioxidants, and phytochemicals that work together to combat inflammation and support overall health. Aim to consume a wide variety of colorful fruits and vegetables to ensure you are getting a diverse array of beneficial compounds.

Leafy greens, such as spinach, kale, and Swiss chard, are particularly potent anti-inflammatory foods. These vegetables are packed with vitamins A, C, and K, as well as minerals like iron and calcium. They also contain powerful antioxidants, such as lutein and zeaxanthin, which help protect cells from oxidative damage and reduce inflammation.

Berries, including blueberries, raspberries, and strawberries, are another excellent choice for an anti-inflammatory diet. These fruits are rich in anthocyanins, a type of flavonoid that gives berries their vibrant color and has been shown to have anti-inflammatory and antioxidant properties. Studies have found that regular consumption of berries may help reduce markers of inflammation, improve insulin sensitivity, and lower the risk of chronic diseases like heart disease and diabetes.

Other anti-inflammatory fruits and vegetables include:

1 Cruciferous vegetables (e.g., broccoli, cauliflower, and Brussels sprouts)

2 Alliums (e.g., garlic, onions, and leeks)

3 Tomatoes

4 Avocados

5 Citrus fruits (e.g., oranges, grapefruits, and lemons)

6 Pomegranates

7 Beets

To maximize the anti-inflammatory benefits of fruits and vegetables, aim to consume a variety of these foods in their whole, minimally processed form. Incorporate them into your meals and snacks throughout the day, and experiment with different preparation methods, such as roasting, sautéing, and blending, to keep things interesting and enjoyable.

Whole grains Whole grains are an important component of an anti-inflammatory diet. Unlike refined grains, which have been stripped of their bran and germ, whole grains retain all three parts of the grain kernel (bran, germ, and endosperm), providing a rich source of fiber, vitamins, minerals, and phytochemicals.

The fiber in whole grains, particularly the soluble fiber, has been shown to have anti-inflammatory effects in the body. Soluble fiber helps feed the beneficial bacteria in the gut, promoting the production of short-chain fatty acids (SCFAs) that have anti-inflammatory properties. Additionally, fiber helps slow down digestion and stabilize blood sugar levels, reducing the risk of insulin resistance and chronic inflammation.

Some of the best whole grains to include in an anti-inflammatory diet are:

1 Oats

2 Brown rice

3 Quinoa

4 Bulgur

5 Barley

6 Millet

7 Sorghum

When selecting whole-grain products, such as bread, pasta, and cereals, be sure to read the ingredient list carefully. Look for items that list a whole grain as the first ingredient and are free from added sugars and artificial additives. Alternatively, you can prepare whole grains at home by cooking them in water or low-sodium broth until tender.

Healthy fats (omega-3s, monounsaturated fats) Healthy fats, particularly omega-3 fatty acids and monounsaturated fats, are essential for reducing inflammation and supporting overall health. These fats help regulate the production of inflammatory compounds in the body and have been linked to a lower risk of chronic diseases like heart disease, stroke, and certain cancers.

Omega-3 fatty acids, specifically eicosapentaenoic acid (EPA) and docosahexaenoic acid (DHA), are potent anti-inflammatory compounds found primarily in fatty fish. These fats help reduce the production of pro-inflammatory cytokines and promote the synthesis of anti-inflammatory mediators called resolvins and protectins. The best sources of EPA and DHA include:

1 Salmon

2 Sardines

3 Mackerel

4 Herring

5 Anchovies

6 Trout

Plant-based sources of omega-3s, such as flaxseeds, chia seeds, and walnuts, contain alpha-linolenic acid (ALA), which the body can convert to EPA and DHA, albeit in small amounts. While these foods are still beneficial, it is important for those following a plant-based diet to consider taking an algae-based omega-3 supplement to ensure adequate intake of EPA and DHA.

Monounsaturated fats, found in foods like olive oil, avocados, and nuts, have also been shown to have anti-inflammatory properties. These fats help reduce LDL ("bad") cholesterol levels and increase HDL ("good") cholesterol levels, which can help lower the risk of heart disease and inflammation. Some of the best sources of monounsaturated fats include:

1 Extra virgin olive oil

2 Avocados

3 Almonds

4 Cashews

5 Pistachios

6 Hazelnuts

7 Macadamia nuts

To incorporate healthy fats into your anti-inflammatory diet, use olive oil as your primary cooking oil, snack on a handful of nuts or seeds, and add sliced avocado to your salads and sandwiches. Remember to consume these fats in moderation, as they are still calorie-dense and can contribute to weight gain if eaten in excess.

Lean proteins Protein is an essential macronutrient that plays a crucial role in building and repairing tissues, producing enzymes and hormones, and supporting immune function. When it comes to an anti-inflammatory diet, focusing on lean, high-quality protein sources is key to reducing inflammation and promoting optimal health.

Some of the best lean protein sources for an anti-inflammatory diet include:

1 Fatty fish (e.g., salmon, sardines, and mackerel)

2 Skinless poultry (e.g., chicken and turkey)

3 Legumes (e.g., beans, lentils, and peas)

4 Tofu and tempeh

5 Greek yogurt

6 Eggs

7 Nuts and seeds

Fatty fish, as mentioned earlier, are an excellent source of omega-3 fatty acids, which have potent anti-inflammatory properties. Aim to consume fatty fish at least twice a week to reap the benefits of these healthy fats.

Legumes are another great option for those following an anti-inflammatory diet. These plant-based proteins are rich in fiber, vitamins, minerals, and phytochemicals that have been shown to have anti-inflammatory effects. Legumes are also low in fat and high in protein, making them a satisfying and nutrient-dense addition to meals and snacks.

When selecting lean proteins, it is important to choose high-quality sources that are minimally processed and free from added hormones and antibiotics. Opt for organic, grass-fed, and pasture-raised options whenever possible, as these animals are typically raised in more humane conditions and may have a more favorable fatty acid profile compared to conventionally raised animals.

Herbs and spices Herbs and spices are not only a great way to add flavor and depth to your meals but also offer a wide range of anti-inflammatory compounds that can help reduce inflammation and support overall health. Many herbs and spices contain potent antioxidants and phytochemicals that have been shown to have anti-inflammatory, antimicrobial, and even anticancer properties.

Some of the best anti-inflammatory herbs and spices to incorporate into your diet include:

1 Turmeric: This bright yellow spice contains curcumin, a powerful anti-inflammatory compound that has been shown to help reduce inflammation, improve brain function, and lower the risk of chronic diseases like heart disease and cancer.

2 Ginger: Ginger contains gingerols and shogaols, which have anti-inflammatory and antioxidant properties. Regular consumption of ginger may help reduce inflammation, alleviate digestive issues, and improve immune function.

3 Garlic: Garlic is rich in sulfur compounds, such as allicin, which have been shown to have anti-inflammatory and antimicrobial effects. Garlic may help lower blood pressure, improve cholesterol levels, and reduce the risk of certain cancers.

4 Cinnamon: This sweet spice contains cinnamaldehyde, a compound that has been shown to have anti-inflammatory and antioxidant properties. Cinnamon may help improve insulin sensitivity, lower blood sugar levels, and reduce the risk of heart disease.

5 Rosemary: Rosemary is rich in rosmarinic acid, a potent anti-inflammatory compound that has been shown to help reduce inflammation, improve brain function, and protect against oxidative stress.

6 Cayenne pepper: Cayenne contains capsaicin, a compound that has been shown to have anti-inflammatory and pain-relieving properties. Capsaicin may help reduce inflammation, improve circulation, and boost metabolism.

7 Sage: Sage contains flavonoids and phenolic acids that have been shown to have anti-inflammatory and antioxidant effects. Sage may help improve brain function, reduce inflammation, and alleviate menopausal symptoms.

To maximize the anti-inflammatory benefits of herbs and spices, aim to incorporate a variety of these flavorful ingredients into your meals and snacks. Use them to season your proteins, vegetables, and whole grains, or steep them in hot water to create anti-inflammatory teas and tonics.

Fermented foods and probiotics Fermented foods and probiotics are another important component of an anti-inflammatory diet. These foods contain beneficial bacteria, known as probiotics, that help support gut health and improve immune function. A healthy gut microbiome is essential for reducing inflammation and preventing chronic diseases.

Some of the best fermented foods and probiotic sources to include in an anti-inflammatory diet are:

1 Yogurt (particularly Greek yogurt and kefir)
2 Sauerkraut
3 Kimchi

4 Miso

5 Tempeh

6 Kombucha

7 Probiotic supplements

Fermented foods are rich in lactic acid bacteria, which help promote the growth of beneficial gut bacteria and improve digestive health. These bacteria also produce short-chain fatty acids (SCFAs), such as butyrate, which have been shown to have anti-inflammatory effects in the gut and throughout the body.

When selecting fermented foods, opt for unpasteurized, traditionally fermented options, as these contain live, active cultures that offer the most significant health benefits. If you are unable to tolerate fermented foods or have a compromised immune system, consider taking a high-quality probiotic supplement to support gut health and reduce inflammation.

Conclusion In this chapter, we have explored the key categories of anti-inflammatory foods to embrace, including fruits and vegetables, whole grains, healthy fats, lean proteins, herbs and spices, and fermented foods and probiotics. By incorporating these nutrient-dense, anti-inflammatory foods into your diet, you can help reduce chronic inflammation, support gut health, and promote overall well-being.

Remember, adopting an anti-inflammatory diet is not about perfection but rather about making consistent, sustainable changes to your eating habits over time. Start by incorporating one or two new anti-inflammatory foods into your diet each week, and gradually build upon these changes as you become more comfortable and confident in your choices.

As with any significant dietary change, it is always best to consult with a healthcare professional or registered dietitian to ensure that your anti-inflammatory diet is balanced, nutritionally adequate, and tailored to your individual needs and preferences. By working with a qualified professional and staying committed to your goals, you can successfully transition to an anti-inflammatory lifestyle and reap the many benefits it has to offer.

LIFESTYLE FACTORS AND INFLAMMATION

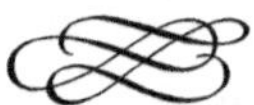

*W*hile adopting an anti-inflammatory diet is a crucial component of reducing chronic inflammation and promoting optimal health, it is essential to recognize that diet is just one piece of the puzzle. Various lifestyle factors, such as physical activity, stress management, sleep, and hydration, also play significant roles in either exacerbating or mitigating inflammation in the body. In this chapter, we will explore the importance of regular exercise, stress management techniques, adequate sleep, staying hydrated, and limiting alcohol consumption in the context of an anti-inflammatory lifestyle.

The importance of regular exercise Regular physical activity is a vital component of an anti-inflammatory lifestyle. Exercise has been shown to have potent anti-inflammatory effects, helping to reduce markers of inflammation, improve insulin sensitivity, and support cardiovascular health. Engaging in regular exercise can also help maintain a healthy weight, which is crucial for reducing inflamma-tion, as excess body fat, particularly visceral fat, is a significant source of pro-inflammatory compounds.

The anti-inflammatory effects of exercise are mediated through several mechanisms. During physical activity, muscles release anti-inflammatory cytokines, such as interleukin-6 (IL-6), which help suppress the production of pro-inflammatory cytokines like tumor necrosis factor-alpha (TNF-α) and interleukin-1 beta (IL-1β). Exercise also helps reduce levels of C-reactive protein (CRP), a marker of systemic inflammation that has been linked to an increased risk of heart disease and other chronic conditions.

In addition to its direct anti-inflammatory effects, regular exercise can also help reduce inflammation indirectly by improving other lifestyle factors. For example, physical activity can help reduce stress, improve sleep quality, and support healthy weight management, all of which contribute to lower levels of inflammation in the body.

To reap the anti-inflammatory benefits of exercise, aim to engage in at least 150 minutes of moderate-intensity aerobic activity or 75 minutes of vigorous-intensity aerobic activity per week, along with two to three sessions of strength training. Some examples of anti-inflammatory exercises include:

1 Brisk walking
2 Jogging or running
3 Swimming
4 Cycling
5 Dancing
6 Yoga
7 Resistance training (e.g., weightlifting, bodyweight exercises)

Remember to start slowly and gradually increase the intensity and duration of your workouts to prevent injury and ensure long-term adherence. If you have a pre-existing health condition or have been sedentary for an extended period, consult with a healthcare professional before starting a new exercise routine.

Stress management techniques Chronic stress is a significant contributor to inflammation in the body. When the body is under stress, it releases cortisol, a hormone that helps mobilize energy and prepare the body for a "fight or flight" response. While this response is essential for short-term survival, chronic activation of the stress response can lead to persistently elevated levels of cortisol, which can promote inflammation and disrupt various physiological processes.

Chronic stress has been linked to an increased risk of numerous health problems, including heart disease, diabetes, autoimmune disorders, and mental health issues like depression and anxiety. To reduce inflammation and support overall health, it is crucial to incorporate stress management techniques into your daily routine.

Some effective stress management techniques include:

1 Mindfulness meditation: Mindfulness involves focusing on the present moment and observing your thoughts and feelings without judgment. Regular mindfulness practice has been shown to reduce stress, improve emotional regulation, and lower levels of pro-inflammatory cytokines.

2 Deep breathing exercises: Deep, diaphragmatic breathing can help activate the parasympathetic nervous system, which promotes relaxation and reduces stress. Try taking slow, deep breaths for several minutes each day to calm your mind and body.

3 Progressive muscle relaxation: This technique involves systematically tensing and relaxing different muscle groups in the body to promote relaxation and reduce tension. Start by tensing and relaxing the muscles in your feet, then move up to your calves, thighs, and so on until you reach your head.

4 Yoga: Yoga combines physical postures, breathing exercises, and meditation to promote relaxation, reduce stress, and improve overall well-being. Regular yoga practice has been shown to reduce markers of inflammation and improve mental health.

5 Spending time in nature: Exposure to nature, such as walking in a park or gardening, has been shown to reduce stress, lower cortisol levels, and improve mood. Aim to spend at least 20-30 minutes in nature each day to reap the stress-reducing benefits.

6 Engaging in hobbies: Participating in enjoyable activities, such as reading, painting, or playing music, can help reduce stress and promote relaxation. Make time for your hobbies regularly to support your mental and emotional well-being.

7 Connecting with others: Strong social connections are essential for managing stress and reducing inflammation. Spend quality time

with friends and family, join a support group, or volunteer in your community to foster a sense of belonging and reduce stress.

By incorporating these stress management techniques into your daily routine, you can help reduce inflammation, improve your overall health, and enhance your quality of life.

Adequate sleep and its impact on inflammation Sleep is a critical component of an anti-inflammatory lifestyle. During sleep, the body undergoes numerous restorative processes, including tissue repair, hormone regulation, and immune system support. Inadequate sleep, both in terms of quantity and quality, has been linked to increased levels of inflammation and a higher risk of chronic diseases.

Studies have shown that individuals who consistently get less than 7-8 hours of sleep per night have higher levels of pro-inflammatory markers, such as C-reactive protein (CRP) and interleukin-6 (IL-6). Lack of sleep has also been associated with an increased risk of obesity, insulin resistance, and cardiovascular disease, all of which are characterized by chronic low-grade inflammation.

To support an anti-inflammatory lifestyle, aim to prioritize sleep and ensure that you are getting enough high-quality rest each night. Some tips for improving sleep quality and reducing inflammation include:

1 Stick to a consistent sleep schedule: Go to bed and wake up at the same time each day, even on weekends, to help regulate your body's internal clock and improve sleep quality.

2 Create a relaxing bedtime routine: Engage in calming activities, such as reading, taking a warm bath, or practicing relaxation techniques, before bed to help signal to your body that it's time to sleep.

3 Optimize your sleep environment: Ensure that your bedroom is dark, quiet, and cool, and invest in a comfortable, supportive mattress and pillows to promote restful sleep.

4 Limit exposure to electronic devices before bed: The blue light emitted by electronic devices can interfere with your body's production of melatonin, a hormone that regulates sleep. Aim to avoid screens for at least an hour before bedtime.

5 Avoid stimulants and large meals close to bedtime: Caffeine,

alcohol, and large, heavy meals can disrupt sleep quality and exacerbate inflammation. Try to avoid these substances and foods for at least 2-3 hours before bed.

6 Engage in regular physical activity: As discussed earlier, regular exercise can help reduce inflammation and improve sleep quality. However, avoid vigorous exercise close to bedtime, as it may interfere with your ability to fall asleep.

7 Manage stress: Chronic stress can disrupt sleep quality and contribute to inflammation. Incorporate stress management techniques, such as mindfulness meditation or deep breathing exercises, into your daily routine to support restful sleep.

By prioritizing sleep and taking steps to improve sleep quality, you can help reduce inflammation, support your immune system, and promote overall health and well-being.

Staying hydrated and limiting alcohol consumption Staying hydrated and limiting alcohol consumption are two additional lifestyle factors that can have a significant impact on inflammation in the body. Proper hydration is essential for maintaining healthy bodily functions, supporting immune system function, and flushing out toxins and waste products that can contribute to inflammation. On the other hand, excessive alcohol consumption has been linked to increased levels of inflammation and a higher risk of chronic diseases.

Water is the best choice for staying hydrated, as it is calorie-free and readily available. Aim to drink at least 8-10 glasses (64-80 ounces) of water per day, and more if you are exercising, living in a hot climate, or experiencing illness. In addition to water, you can also stay hydrated by consuming water-rich foods, such as fruits and vegetables, and unsweetened herbal teas.

Limiting alcohol consumption is crucial for reducing inflammation and supporting overall health. While moderate alcohol consumption (defined as up to one drink per day for women and up to two drinks per day for men) has been associated with some potential health benefits, such as a reduced risk of heart disease, excessive alcohol intake can have detrimental effects on the body.

Alcohol has been shown to disrupt the balance of gut bacteria, leading to increased intestinal permeability (leaky gut) and systemic inflammation. It can also interfere with the body's ability to absorb and utilize essential nutrients, such as vitamins and minerals, which are necessary for maintaining a healthy immune system and reducing inflammation.

Moreover, alcohol is a significant source of empty calories and can contribute to weight gain, which is a risk factor for chronic inflammation. Excessive alcohol consumption has also been linked to an increased risk of liver damage, certain cancers, and mental health issues like depression and anxiety.

To minimize the inflammatory effects of alcohol, consider the following tips:

1 Limit your intake: If you choose to drink, do so in moderation, and avoid binge drinking (defined as four or more drinks for women and five or more drinks for men in a single occasion).

2 Choose low-sugar options: Mixers like soda, tonic water, and fruit juices can add significant amounts of sugar to alcoholic beverages, which can further exacerbate inflammation. Opt for low-sugar options, such as seltzer water or fresh lime juice, instead.

3 Alternate with water: When drinking alcohol, alternate each alcoholic beverage with a glass of water to help stay hydrated and slow your alcohol consumption.

4 Avoid drinking on an empty stomach: Consuming alcohol on an empty stomach can lead to more rapid absorption and increase the risk of inflammation and other negative health effects. If you choose to drink, do so with a meal or snack that contains protein, healthy fats, and fiber to slow alcohol absorption.

5 Take breaks from alcohol: Consider taking regular breaks from alcohol consumption, such as abstaining for a week or month, to give your body a chance to recover and reduce overall inflammation.

By staying hydrated and limiting alcohol consumption, you can support your body's natural anti-inflammatory processes and promote overall health and well-being.

Conclusion In this chapter, we have explored the various lifestyle factors that can impact inflammation in the body, including the importance of regular exercise, stress management techniques, adequate sleep, staying hydrated, and limiting alcohol consumption. By incorporating these lifestyle strategies into your daily routine, alongside an anti-inflammatory diet, you can take a comprehensive approach to reducing chronic inflammation and promoting optimal health.

Remember, making lasting lifestyle changes takes time, patience, and self-compassion. Start by setting small, achievable goals for yourself, and celebrate your progress along the way. If you encounter setbacks or challenges, don't be discouraged – simply regroup and refocus on your goals, and seek support from friends, family, or a healthcare professional when needed.

By prioritizing self-care and making consistent, sustainable changes to your lifestyle, you can create a strong foundation for long-term health and well-being. In the next chapter, we will delve into the practical aspects of implementing an anti-inflammatory diet and lifestyle, including tips for meal planning, dining out, and staying motivated on your journey toward optimal health.

IMPLEMENTING THE ANTI-INFLAMMATORY DIET

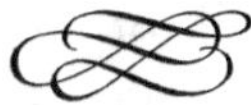

Transitioning to an anti-inflammatory diet and lifestyle can be a significant change, and it's essential to approach it with a well-thought-out plan to ensure long-term success. In this chapter, we will discuss strategies for gradually transitioning to the diet, dealing with cravings and temptations, navigating eating out and social situations, tracking your progress and symptoms, and staying motivated while overcoming obstacles.

Gradual transition to the diet When embarking on an anti-inflammatory diet, it's crucial to make gradual changes rather than attempting a complete overhaul overnight. This approach allows your body and mind to adapt to the new way of eating, increasing the likelihood of long-term adherence. Here are some tips for gradually transitioning to an anti-inflammatory diet:

1 Start by adding, not subtracting: Begin by incorporating more anti-inflammatory foods into your diet, such as fruits, vegetables, whole grains, and healthy fats, without focusing on eliminating less healthy options. As you become more comfortable with these new foods, you'll naturally start to crowd out the less nutritious choices.

2 Make one change at a time: Each week, set a goal to make one significant change to your diet, such as replacing refined grains with

whole grains or swapping sugary snacks for fruit. By focusing on one change at a time, you'll be less likely to feel overwhelmed and more likely to stick with your new habits.

3 Plan and prepare: Set aside time each week to plan your meals and snacks, and prepare ingredients in advance. Having a well-stocked kitchen and ready-to-eat, anti-inflammatory options on hand will make it easier to make healthy choices when hunger strikes.

4 Be patient with yourself: Remember that adopting an anti-inflammatory diet is a journey, not a destination. There will be ups and downs along the way, and that's okay. Be patient with yourself, celebrate your successes, and learn from your setbacks.

Dealing with cravings and temptations As you transition to an anti-inflammatory diet, it's normal to experience cravings for less healthy foods, especially those that you may have relied on for comfort or convenience in the past. Here are some strategies for dealing with cravings and temptations:

1 Identify your triggers: Take note of the situations, emotions, or times of day when cravings tend to strike. By becoming more aware of your triggers, you can develop a plan to cope with them in a healthy way.

2 Practice mindful eating: When a craving hits, take a moment to pause and check in with yourself. Are you truly hungry, or are you experiencing an emotional or habitual response? If you decide to indulge in a less healthy option, do so mindfully, savoring each bite and paying attention to how the food makes you feel.

3 Find healthy substitutes: Stock your kitchen with healthy, anti-inflammatory alternatives to your favorite treats. For example, if you crave something sweet, reach for a piece of fruit or a small square of dark chocolate instead of processed candy.

4 Distract yourself: When a craving feels overwhelming, try engaging in an activity that takes your mind off of food, such as going for a walk, reading a book, or calling a friend. Often, cravings will pass if you give them time and distance.

5 Practice self-compassion: If you do give in to a craving, don't beat yourself up about it. Treat yourself with kindness and under-

standing, and remember that one less-than-perfect choice doesn't define your entire journey. Simply get back on track with your next meal or snack.

Eating out and social situations Navigating eating out and social situations can be challenging when following an anti-inflammatory diet, but with a bit of planning and assertiveness, you can stay on track while still enjoying time with friends and family. Here are some tips:

1 Research menus ahead of time: If you know where you'll be dining out, look up the menu online and identify the most anti-inflammatory options. Many restaurants now offer allergen and ingredient information, making it easier to make informed choices.

2 Don't be afraid to make special requests: When ordering, ask for modifications to suit your needs, such as requesting steamed vegetables instead of fries or asking for sauces and dressings on the side. Most restaurants are happy to accommodate special dietary needs.

3 Bring your own dish to social gatherings: If you're attending a potluck or party, offer to bring an anti-inflammatory dish that you know you can enjoy. This ensures that you'll have at least one healthy option available, and you may even inspire others to try something new.

4 Focus on social connection: Remember that social gatherings are about more than just food. Shift your focus to enjoying the company of others and engaging in meaningful conversations, rather than fixating on what you can or can't eat.

5 Communicate your needs: If you're dining at the home of a friend or family member, let them know ahead of time about your dietary preferences. Offer to bring a dish or suggest anti-inflammatory options that they can easily incorporate into the menu.

Tracking your progress and symptoms Keeping track of your progress and symptoms can be a valuable tool for staying motivated and identifying patterns between your diet and overall health. Here are some ways to track your anti-inflammatory journey:

1 Keep a food and symptom journal: Record what you eat each day, along with any symptoms you experience, such as pain, fatigue,

or digestive issues. Over time, you may start to notice connections between certain foods and how you feel.

2 Monitor your weight and body measurements: While weight loss may not be the primary goal of an anti-inflammatory diet, it can be a helpful indicator of progress. Take measurements of your waist, hips, and other areas of concern to track changes over time.

3 Assess your energy levels and mood: Pay attention to your overall sense of well-being, including your energy levels, mood, and sleep quality. Note any improvements or changes as you continue on your anti-inflammatory journey.

4 Get regular check-ups and blood work: Work with your health-care provider to monitor markers of inflammation, such as C-reactive protein (CRP) and erythrocyte sedimentation rate (ESR). Regular check-ups can help you track your progress and make adjustments to your diet and lifestyle as needed.

Staying motivated and overcoming obstacles Adopting an anti-inflammatory diet and lifestyle is a long-term commitment, and it's normal to face challenges and obstacles along the way. Here are some strategies for staying motivated and overcoming setbacks:

1 Set realistic goals and celebrate your progress: Break your larger goals into smaller, achievable milestones, and celebrate each victory along the way. Acknowledging your progress, no matter how small, can help keep you motivated and on track.

2 Find a support system: Surround yourself with people who support your anti-inflammatory journey, whether it's friends and family members who share your goals or an online community of like-minded individuals. Having a strong support system can provide encouragement, accountability, and inspiration.

3 Focus on how you feel, not just how you look: While physical changes can be rewarding, remember that the primary goal of an anti-inflammatory diet is to improve your overall health and well-being. Pay attention to how your body feels, and let that be your guide.

4 Be prepared for setbacks: Setbacks and slip-ups are a normal part of any lifestyle change. When they happen, don't dwell on them

or let them derail your progress. Instead, use them as learning opportunities and get back on track with your next meal or snack.

5 Continuously educate yourself: Stay informed about the latest research and insights related to anti-inflammatory living. Read books, articles, and blogs, listen to podcasts, and attend workshops or seminars to deepen your understanding and stay inspired.

By implementing these strategies and maintaining a positive, patient mindset, you can successfully navigate the challenges of adopting an anti-inflammatory diet and lifestyle, ultimately creating a foundation for long-term health and well-being.

RECIPES FOR EVERY MEAL

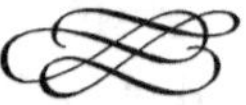

*N*ow that you have a solid understanding of the principles behind an anti-inflammatory diet and lifestyle, it's time to put that knowledge into practice with delicious, nourishing recipes for every meal. In this chapter, we'll explore a variety of anti-inflammatory breakfast, lunch, dinner, snack, dessert, smoothie, and beverage recipes that will help you stay on track and enjoy the journey to better health.

Breakfast Recipes Starting your day with a nutritious, anti-inflammatory breakfast sets the stage for better choices throughout the day. These recipes are packed with fiber, healthy fats, and antioxidants to keep you feeling satisfied and energized.

1 Coconut Chia Seed Pudding Ingredients:
- 1/2 cup chia seeds
- 2 cups unsweetened coconut milk
- 1 tsp vanilla extract
- 1 tbsp maple syrup or honey (optional)
- 1/2 cup mixed berries
- 1/4 cup unsweetened shredded coconut

Instructions:

1 In a large bowl, whisk together the chia seeds, coconut milk, vanilla extract, and sweetener (if using) until well combined.

2 Cover the bowl with plastic wrap and refrigerate for at least 2 hours or overnight, stirring occasionally to prevent clumping.

3 When ready to serve, divide the pudding into bowls and top with mixed berries and shredded coconut.

4 Avocado and Egg Toast Ingredients:

• 2 slices whole-grain bread

• 1 ripe avocado, mashed

• 2 eggs

• 1/4 tsp paprika

• Salt and pepper to taste

Instructions:

1 Toast the bread until golden brown.

2 In a small bowl, mash the avocado with a fork and spread it evenly on the toast.

3 In a non-stick skillet, cook the eggs to your liking (scrambled, poached, or fried).

4 Place the cooked eggs on top of the avocado toast, and sprinkle with paprika, salt, and pepper.

5 Anti-Inflammatory Smoothie Bowl Ingredients:

• 1 frozen banana

• 1 cup frozen mixed berries

• 1/2 cup unsweetened almond milk

• 1 tbsp chia seeds

• 1 tbsp almond butter

• 1/2 tsp ground turmeric

• 1/4 tsp ground ginger

• Toppings: sliced almonds, fresh berries, and unsweetened shredded coconut

Instructions:

1 In a blender, combine the frozen banana, mixed berries, almond milk, chia seeds, almond butter, turmeric, and ginger. Blend until smooth and creamy.

2 Pour the smoothie into a bowl and add your desired toppings.

Lunch Recipes These anti-inflammatory lunch recipes are perfect for busy weekdays when you need something quick, satisfying, and nutritious.

1 Quinoa and Veggie Stir-Fry Ingredients:
• 1 cup cooked quinoa
• 1 tbsp coconut oil
• 1 small onion, diced
• 2 garlic cloves, minced
• 1 red bell pepper, sliced
• 1 cup broccoli florets
• 1 cup sliced mushrooms
• 1 tbsp grated ginger
• 2 tbsp low-sodium soy sauce
• 1 tbsp sesame oil
• Salt and pepper to taste
Instructions:
1 In a large skillet or wok, heat the coconut oil over medium heat.
2 Add the onion and garlic, and sauté until fragrant, about 2 minutes.
3 Add the bell pepper, broccoli, and mushrooms, and stir-fry for 5-7 minutes or until the vegetables are tender-crisp.
4 Stir in the cooked quinoa, ginger, soy sauce, and sesame oil. Season with salt and pepper to taste.
5 Cook for an additional 2-3 minutes, stirring occasionally, until the quinoa is heated through.
6 Mediterranean Tuna Salad Ingredients:
• 1 can (5 oz) wild-caught tuna, drained
• 1/4 cup diced red onion
• 1/4 cup diced cucumber
• 1/4 cup diced cherry tomatoes
• 2 tbsp chopped Kalamata olives
• 2 tbsp extra-virgin olive oil
• 1 tbsp freshly squeezed lemon juice
• 1/4 tsp dried oregano
• Salt and pepper to taste

• Mixed greens for serving

Instructions:

1 In a medium bowl, combine the tuna, red onion, cucumber, cherry tomatoes, and Kalamata olives.

2 In a small bowl, whisk together the olive oil, lemon juice, oregano, salt, and pepper.

3 Pour the dressing over the tuna mixture and toss gently to coat.

4 Serve the tuna salad over a bed of mixed greens.

5 Lentil and Vegetable Soup Ingredients:

• 1 tbsp extra-virgin olive oil
• 1 medium onion, diced
• 2 carrots, diced
• 2 celery stalks, diced
• 3 garlic cloves, minced
• 1 tsp ground cumin
• 1 tsp ground coriander
• 1 cup dried green or brown lentils, rinsed
• 4 cups low-sodium vegetable broth
• 1 can (14.5 oz) diced tomatoes
• 1 bay leaf
• 2 cups baby spinach
• Salt and pepper to taste

Instructions:

1 In a large pot, heat the olive oil over medium heat. Add the onion, carrots, and celery, and sauté until the vegetables are softened, about 5 minutes.

2 Add the garlic, cumin, and coriander, and cook for an additional 1-2 minutes, until fragrant.

3 Stir in the lentils, vegetable broth, diced tomatoes, and bay leaf. Bring the soup to a boil, then reduce the heat and simmer for 25-30 minutes or until the lentils are tender.

4 Remove the bay leaf and stir in the baby spinach until wilted.

5 Season with salt and pepper to taste before serving.

Dinner Recipes These anti-inflammatory dinner recipes are

perfect for gathering friends and family around the table for a nourishing, delicious meal.

1 Baked Salmon with Asparagus and Sweet Potato Ingredients:
• 4 wild-caught salmon fillets (4-6 oz each)
• 1 lb asparagus, trimmed
• 2 medium sweet potatoes, diced
• 2 tbsp extra-virgin olive oil
• 1 tsp dried dill
• 1 tsp garlic powder
• Salt and pepper to taste
• Lemon wedges for serving
Instructions:
1 Preheat the oven to 400°F (200°C).
2 On a large baking sheet, arrange the salmon fillets, asparagus, and diced sweet potatoes in a single layer.
3 Drizzle the olive oil over the salmon, asparagus, and sweet potatoes. Sprinkle with dill, garlic powder, salt, and pepper.
4 Bake for 15-20 minutes or until the salmon is cooked through and the vegetables are tender.
5 Serve with lemon wedges on the side.
6 Slow Cooker Turmeric Chicken Ingredients:
• 1 tbsp coconut oil
• 1 medium onion, diced
• 4 garlic cloves, minced
• 1 tbsp grated ginger
• 1 tbsp ground turmeric
• 1 tsp ground cumin
• 1/2 tsp ground cinnamon
• 1/4 tsp cayenne pepper (optional)
• 1 can (14.5 oz) diced tomatoes
• 1 cup low-sodium chicken broth
• 2 lbs boneless, skinless chicken breasts or thighs
• 1 can (13.5 oz) full-fat coconut milk
• Salt and pepper to taste
• Fresh cilantro for garnish

Instructions:

1 In a large skillet, heat the coconut oil over medium heat. Add the onion and sauté until softened, about 5 minutes.

2 Add the garlic, ginger, turmeric, cumin, cinnamon, and cayenne (if using), and cook for an additional 1-2 minutes, until fragrant.

3 Transfer the onion mixture to a slow cooker. Add the diced tomatoes, chicken broth, and chicken. Stir to combine.

4 Cover and cook on low for 6-8 hours or on high for 3-4 hours, until the chicken is tender and cooked through.

5 Shred the chicken with two forks and stir in the coconut milk. Season with salt and pepper to taste.

6 Serve over brown rice or quinoa, garnished with fresh cilantro.

7 Quinoa Stuffed Bell Peppers Ingredients:

- 4 large bell peppers (any color), halved and seeded
- 1 cup uncooked quinoa, rinsed
- 1 tbsp extra-virgin olive oil
- 1 small onion, diced
- 2 garlic cloves, minced
- 1 lb lean ground turkey
- 1 tsp ground cumin
- 1 tsp smoked paprika
- 1 can (14.5 oz) diced tomatoes
- 1/2 cup low-sodium chicken broth
- 1/4 cup chopped fresh parsley
- Salt and pepper to taste

Instructions:

1 Preheat the oven to 375°F (190°C).

2 Place the bell pepper halves in a baking dish, cut-side up. Set aside.

3 In a medium saucepan, cook the quinoa according to package instructions.

4 In a large skillet, heat the olive oil over medium heat. Add the onion and sauté until softened, about 5 minutes.

5 Add the garlic and ground turkey to the skillet. Cook, breaking

up the turkey with a wooden spoon, until browned and cooked through.

6 Stir in the cumin, smoked paprika, diced tomatoes, chicken broth, and cooked quinoa. Simmer for 5 minutes, stirring occasionally.

7 Remove the skillet from the heat and stir in the chopped parsley. Season with salt and pepper to taste.

8 Spoon the quinoa mixture into the bell pepper halves. Cover the baking dish with foil.

9 Bake for 30-35 minutes or until the bell peppers are tender. Remove the foil for the last 5 minutes of baking.

Snacks and Desserts These anti-inflammatory snacks and desserts are perfect for satisfying your cravings while still nourishing your body.

1 Roasted Spiced Chickpeas Ingredients:
• 1 can (15 oz) chickpeas, drained and rinsed
• 1 tbsp extra-virgin olive oil
• 1 tsp ground cumin
• 1 tsp smoked paprika
• 1/2 tsp garlic powder
• 1/4 tsp cayenne pepper (optional)
• Salt and pepper to taste
Instructions:
1 Preheat the oven to 400°F (200°C).
2 Pat the chickpeas dry with a paper towel and remove any loose skins.

3 In a medium bowl, toss the chickpeas with olive oil, cumin, smoked paprika, garlic powder, cayenne (if using), salt, and pepper.

4 Spread the chickpeas in a single layer on a baking sheet.

5 Roast for 30-35 minutes, stirring halfway through, until crispy and golden brown.

6 Let cool before serving.

7 Dark Chocolate Avocado Mousse Ingredients:
• 2 ripe avocados, pitted and peeled
• 1/2 cup unsweetened cocoa powder

- 1/4 cup pure maple syrup
- 1/4 cup unsweetened almond milk
- 1 tsp vanilla extract
- Pinch of salt
- Fresh berries for garnish

Instructions:

1 In a food processor or blender, combine the avocados, cocoa powder, maple syrup, almond milk, vanilla extract, and salt.

2 Process until smooth and creamy, scraping down the sides as needed.

3 Spoon the mousse into individual serving dishes and refrigerate for at least 30 minutes before serving.

4 Garnish with fresh berries before serving.

5 Turmeric Spiced Nuts Ingredients:

- 2 cups raw mixed nuts (almonds, cashews, pecans, etc.)
- 1 tbsp extra-virgin olive oil
- 1 tsp ground turmeric
- 1/2 tsp ground cinnamon
- 1/4 tsp ground ginger
- 1/4 tsp cayenne pepper (optional)
- 1 tbsp pure maple syrup
- Salt to taste

Instructions:

1 Preheat the oven to 300°F (150°C).

2 In a medium bowl, combine the mixed nuts, olive oil, turmeric, cinnamon, ginger, cayenne (if using), maple syrup, and salt. Toss until the nuts are evenly coated.

3 Spread the nuts in a single layer on a baking sheet lined with parchment paper.

4 Bake for 20-25 minutes, stirring halfway through, until the nuts are lightly toasted and fragrant.

5 Let cool completely before serving.

Smoothies and Beverages These anti-inflammatory smoothies and beverages are perfect for hydrating and nourishing your body while providing a delicious treat.

1 Green Detox Smoothie Ingredients:
• 1 cup baby spinach
• 1 small cucumber, chopped
• 1 small green apple, cored and chopped
• 1/2 lemon, juiced
• 1/2 inch fresh ginger, peeled and grated
• 1 tbsp chia seeds
• 1 cup unsweetened coconut water
Instructions:
1 In a blender, combine the spinach, cucumber, apple, lemon juice, ginger, chia seeds, and coconut water.
2 Blend until smooth and creamy.
3 Pour into a glass and serve immediately.
4 Turmeric Latte (Golden Milk) Ingredients:
• 1 cup unsweetened almond milk
• 1 tsp ground turmeric
• 1/4 tsp ground cinnamon
• 1/8 tsp ground ginger
• Pinch of black pepper
• 1 tsp pure maple syrup or honey (optional)
Instructions:
1 In a small saucepan, combine the almond milk, turmeric, cinnamon, ginger, and black pepper.
2 Heat over medium heat, whisking constantly, until the mixture is hot and frothy (do not boil).
3 Remove from heat and stir in the maple syrup or honey, if using.
4 Pour into a mug and serve immediately.
5 Watermelon and Mint Cooler Ingredients:
• 4 cups seedless watermelon, cubed
• 1/4 cup fresh mint leaves
• 1 lime, juiced
• 1 cup ice cubes
Instructions:
1 In a blender, combine the watermelon cubes, mint leaves, and lime juice.

2 Blend until smooth.

3 Add the ice cubes and blend until slushy.

4 Pour into glasses and serve immediately.

These anti-inflammatory recipes for every meal demonstrate that eating a nutritious, inflammation-fighting diet can be delicious and enjoyable. By incorporating a variety of colorful fruits and vegetables, whole grains, lean proteins, and healthy fats into your meals and snacks, you can support your body's natural anti-inflammatory processes and promote optimal health.

Remember, the key to success with any dietary change is to start small and make sustainable, long-term shifts in your eating habits. Don't feel pressured to overhaul your entire diet overnight. Instead, focus on incorporating one or two new anti-inflammatory recipes each week, and gradually build upon your repertoire of healthy, delicious meals.

As you continue on your anti-inflammatory journey, keep an open mind and be willing to experiment with new ingredients and flavor combinations. You may be surprised at how satisfying and enjoyable an anti-inflammatory diet can be, and how much better

ADDRESSING SPECIFIC HEALTH CONCERNS

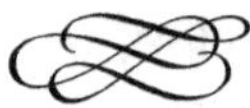

An anti-inflammatory diet can be a powerful tool for managing and preventing various health conditions. By reducing chronic inflammation in the body, this way of eating can help alleviate symptoms, slow disease progression, and improve overall quality of life. In this chapter, we will explore how an anti-inflammatory diet can be tailored to address specific health concerns, including arthritis, autoimmune disorders, heart health, brain health, and skin health.

Anti-inflammatory diet for arthritis Arthritis is a general term for joint inflammation, which can cause pain, stiffness, and swelling in the affected areas. The two most common types of arthritis are osteoarthritis and rheumatoid arthritis. While osteoarthritis is often associated with wear and tear on the joints, rheumatoid arthritis is an autoimmune disorder that causes the body's immune system to attack healthy joint tissue.

An anti-inflammatory diet can be particularly beneficial for individuals with arthritis, as it helps reduce inflammation in the body and alleviate joint pain and stiffness. Here are some specific dietary recommendations for managing arthritis:

1 Increase omega-3 fatty acids: Omega-3s, found in fatty fish like

salmon, sardines, and mackerel, as well as in flaxseeds, chia seeds, and walnuts, have potent anti-inflammatory properties that can help reduce joint inflammation and pain.

2 Limit omega-6 fatty acids: While some omega-6 fatty acids are essential for health, consuming too many can promote inflammation. Reduce your intake of processed foods, fried foods, and vegetable oils high in omega-6s, such as soybean, corn, and sunflower oils.

3 Incorporate turmeric: Turmeric contains curcumin, a powerful anti-inflammatory compound that has been shown to reduce joint pain and stiffness in individuals with arthritis. Add turmeric to your meals or consider taking a curcumin supplement.

4 Eat plenty of fruits and vegetables: Fruits and vegetables are rich in antioxidants and phytochemicals that help combat inflammation in the body. Aim for a variety of colorful produce to ensure you're getting a wide range of beneficial compounds.

5 Choose whole grains: Whole grains, such as brown rice, quinoa, and whole wheat, are high in fiber and nutrients that can help reduce inflammation. Avoid refined grains, which can promote inflammation.

6 Limit added sugars and processed foods: Added sugars and processed foods can trigger inflammation in the body, exacerbating arthritis symptoms. Choose whole, minimally processed foods whenever possible.

By following these dietary guidelines, individuals with arthritis can help manage their symptoms, reduce pain and stiffness, and improve their overall quality of life.

Anti-inflammatory diet for autoimmune disorders Autoimmune disorders occur when the body's immune system mistakenly attacks healthy cells and tissues, leading to chronic inflammation and a variety of symptoms. Examples of autoimmune disorders include rheumatoid arthritis, lupus, multiple sclerosis, and inflammatory bowel disease (IBD).

An anti-inflammatory diet can be an essential component of managing autoimmune disorders, as it helps regulate the immune system and reduce inflammation in the body. Here are some specific dietary recommendations for individuals with autoimmune disorders:

1 Identify and eliminate trigger foods: Some foods, such as gluten, dairy, soy, and eggs, can trigger inflammation and exacerbate autoimmune symptoms in certain individuals. Consider working with a healthcare professional to identify your specific trigger foods and eliminate them from your diet.

2 Focus on nutrient-dense foods: Nutrient-dense foods, such as fruits, vegetables, whole grains, lean proteins, and healthy fats, provide the body with the vitamins, minerals, and antioxidants it needs to function optimally and regulate inflammation.

3 Incorporate fermented foods: Fermented foods, such as sauerkraut, kimchi, and kefir, contain beneficial bacteria that support gut health and immune function. A healthy gut microbiome is essential for regulating inflammation and managing autoimmune disorders.

4 Consider an elimination diet: An elimination diet involves removing potentially problematic foods from your diet for a period of time, then reintroducing them one by one to identify which foods trigger symptoms. This can be a helpful tool for identifying specific dietary triggers and creating a personalized anti-inflammatory diet plan.

5 Manage stress: Chronic stress can exacerbate inflammation and autoimmune symptoms. Incorporate stress-reducing practices, such as meditation, deep breathing, and gentle exercise, into your daily routine to help manage stress and support overall health.

By following an anti-inflammatory diet and making lifestyle changes to support immune function and reduce inflammation, individuals with autoimmune disorders can better manage their symptoms and improve their quality of life.

Anti-inflammatory diet for heart health Heart disease is a leading cause of death worldwide, and chronic inflammation plays a significant role in its development and progression. An anti-inflammatory diet can be a powerful tool for promoting heart health and reducing the risk of cardiovascular disease.

Here are some specific dietary recommendations for supporting heart health:

1 Embrace healthy fats: Healthy fats, such as those found in olive oil, avocados, nuts, and fatty fish, help reduce inflammation and support heart health. Replace saturated and trans fats with these heart-healthy alternatives.

2 Increase fiber intake: Soluble fiber, found in foods like oats, beans, and fruits, helps lower cholesterol levels and reduce inflammation in the body. Aim for at least 25-30 grams of fiber per day.

3 Limit red and processed meats: Red and processed meats, such as beef, pork, and deli meats, are high in saturated fat and have been linked to increased inflammation and heart disease risk. Choose lean proteins, such as fish, poultry, and plant-based options, instead.

4 Reduce sodium intake: Excess sodium can contribute to high blood pressure, a major risk factor for heart disease. Limit processed foods, which are often high in sodium, and use herbs and spices to flavor your meals instead of salt.

5 Incorporate heart-healthy foods: Certain foods, such as leafy greens, berries, dark chocolate, and green tea, are particularly beneficial for heart health due to their high content of antioxidants and anti-inflammatory compounds. Include these foods in your diet regularly.

6 Limit alcohol consumption: While moderate alcohol consumption (one drink per day for women, two for men) has been associated with some heart health benefits, excessive alcohol intake can increase inflammation and contribute to heart disease risk. If you choose to drink, do so in moderation.

By adopting an anti-inflammatory diet and making heart-healthy lifestyle choices, such as regular exercise and stress management, individuals can reduce their risk of heart disease and promote overall cardiovascular health.

Anti-inflammatory diet for brain health The brain is particularly vulnerable to the effects of chronic inflammation, which has been linked to a variety of neurological and mental health disorders, including depression, anxiety, and neurodegenerative diseases like

Alzheimer's and Parkinson's. An anti-inflammatory diet can help protect brain health and reduce the risk of these conditions.

Here are some specific dietary recommendations for promoting brain health:

1 Prioritize omega-3 fatty acids: Omega-3s, particularly DHA and EPA found in fatty fish, are essential for brain function and have been shown to reduce inflammation and support cognitive health. Aim to consume fatty fish at least twice a week, or consider taking a high-quality omega-3 supplement.

2 Incorporate antioxidant-rich foods: Antioxidants help protect the brain from oxidative stress and inflammation. Include plenty of colorful fruits and vegetables, such as berries, leafy greens, and cruciferous vegetables, in your diet to ensure a high intake of antioxidants.

3 Choose complex carbohydrates: Complex carbohydrates, such as those found in whole grains, legumes, and vegetables, provide steady energy for the brain and help regulate blood sugar levels. Avoid refined carbohydrates and added sugars, which can promote inflammation and negatively impact brain health.

4 Include healthy fats: In addition to omega-3s, other healthy fats, such as those found in avocados, nuts, and seeds, support brain function and help reduce inflammation. Incorporate these healthy fats into your meals and snacks regularly.

5 Limit processed and fried foods: Processed and fried foods are often high in unhealthy fats and added sugars, which can promote inflammation and negatively impact brain health. Choose whole, minimally processed foods whenever possible.

6 Stay hydrated: Proper hydration is essential for optimal brain function. Aim to drink at least 8 glasses of water per day, and limit sugary and caffeinated beverages, which can have a dehydrating effect.

In addition to following an anti-inflammatory diet, engaging in regular exercise, getting adequate sleep, and managing stress are all important for promoting brain health and reducing the risk of neurological and mental health disorders.

Anti-inflammatory diet for skin health The skin is the body's largest organ and is often a visible reflection of overall health and well-being. Chronic inflammation can contribute to a variety of skin conditions, such as acne, eczema, and psoriasis, as well as premature aging. An anti-inflammatory diet can help support skin health and reduce the risk of these conditions.

Here are some specific dietary recommendations for promoting skin health:

1 Stay hydrated: Proper hydration is essential for maintaining healthy, supple skin. Drink plenty of water throughout the day and limit dehydrating beverages, such as alcohol and caffeine.

2 Eat plenty of fruits and vegetables: Fruits and vegetables are rich in antioxidants, vitamins, and minerals that support skin health and help protect against sun damage and premature aging. Aim for a variety of colorful produce to ensure a wide range of beneficial compounds.

3 Include healthy fats: Healthy fats, such as those found in avocados, nuts, seeds, and fatty fish, are essential for maintaining healthy skin cell membranes and reducing inflammation. Incorporate these healthy fats into your meals and snacks regularly.

4 Limit added sugars and processed foods: Added sugars and processed foods can promote inflammation and contribute to skin problems like acne and premature aging. Choose whole, minimally processed foods whenever possible.

5 Consider probiotic-rich foods: Probiotic-rich foods, such as yogurt, kefir, and fermented vegetables, support gut health and may help reduce inflammation in the skin. Include these foods in your diet regularly.

6 Protect your skin from the inside out: In addition to following an anti-inflammatory diet, protect your skin from the outside by wearing broad-spectrum sunscreen, avoiding excessive sun exposure, and not smoking.

Remember, the health of your skin is a reflection of your overall health and well-being. By adopting an anti-inflammatory diet and making lifestyle choices that support skin health, you can help keep your skin looking and feeling its best.

Conclusion An anti-inflammatory diet can be a powerful tool for addressing specific health concerns, including arthritis, autoimmune disorders, heart health, brain health, and skin health. By reducing chronic inflammation in the body, this way of eating can help alleviate symptoms, slow disease progression, and improve overall quality of life.

While the general principles of an anti-inflammatory diet remain consistent across different health concerns, there are specific dietary recommendations that can be particularly beneficial for each condition. By tailoring your anti-inflammatory diet to your unique health needs and working with a healthcare professional to create a personalized plan, you can maximize the potential benefits of this way of eating.

It's important to remember that an anti-inflammatory diet is just one component of a healthy lifestyle. Regular exercise, stress management, adequate sleep, and other healthy habits all play a role in reducing inflammation and promoting optimal health and well-being.

As with any dietary change, it's essential to be patient and consistent when adopting an anti-inflammatory diet. It may take time to see the full benefits, but by making small, sustainable changes over time, you can create lasting habits that support your health and well-being for years to come.

If you are dealing with a specific health concern and are interested in using an anti-inflammatory diet to manage your symptoms and improve your quality of life, be sure to work with a qualified healthcare professional who can provide personalized guidance and support. With the right tools and resources, an anti-inflammatory diet can be a valuable addition to your overall health and wellness plan.

LONG-TERM SUCCESS AND MAINTENANCE

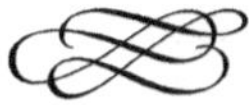

Adopting an anti-inflammatory diet and lifestyle can be a transformative experience, leading to significant improvements in health, well-being, and quality of life. However, the true challenge lies in maintaining these positive changes over the long term. In this final chapter, we will explore strategies for staying committed to the anti-inflammatory lifestyle, customizing the diet to your individual needs, reintroducing foods and monitoring reactions, continuing to learn and stay informed, and celebrating your progress and health improvements.

Staying committed to the anti-inflammatory lifestyle Making lasting changes to your diet and lifestyle requires dedication, persistence, and a strong sense of purpose. Here are some tips for staying committed to the anti-inflammatory lifestyle:

1 Set clear goals: Define your reasons for adopting an anti-inflammatory diet and lifestyle, and set clear, achievable goals that align with your values and priorities. Write these goals down and refer to them regularly to stay motivated and on track.

2 Create a support system: Surround yourself with people who support your health and wellness goals, whether it's friends, family members, or a community of like-minded individuals. Having a

strong support system can provide encouragement, accountability, and motivation when you need it most.

3 Make it a family affair: Involve your family in your anti-inflammatory lifestyle by preparing healthy meals together, engaging in physical activity as a group, and supporting one another's wellness goals. When everyone is on board, it becomes easier to maintain healthy habits long-term.

4 Plan and prepare: Set aside time each week to plan your meals, grocery shop, and prepare healthy snacks and dishes in advance. Having a well-stocked kitchen and ready-to-eat options on hand makes it easier to stick to your anti-inflammatory diet, even when life gets busy.

5 Practice self-compassion: Remember that perfection is not the goal, and it's okay to have occasional setbacks or indulgences. Treat yourself with kindness and understanding, and focus on progress rather than perfection.

6 Celebrate your successes: Acknowledge and celebrate your progress and successes along the way, no matter how small they may seem. Recognizing your achievements can help keep you motivated and committed to your anti-inflammatory lifestyle.

By implementing these strategies and making your anti-inflammatory diet and lifestyle a priority, you can increase your chances of long-term success and reap the many benefits of this healthy way of living.

Customizing the diet to your needs While the general principles of an anti-inflammatory diet remain consistent, it's important to remember that everyone is unique and may have different nutritional needs and preferences. Customizing your anti-inflammatory diet to your individual needs can help ensure long-term success and satisfaction.

Here are some factors to consider when tailoring your anti-inflammatory diet:

1 Food sensitivities and allergies: If you have any known food sensitivities or allergies, it's essential to avoid those foods and focus on incorporating safe, nourishing alternatives into your diet.

2 Health conditions: Certain health conditions may require specific dietary modifications. For example, individuals with celiac disease must avoid gluten, while those with diabetes may need to pay closer attention to their carbohydrate intake. Work with a healthcare professional to determine any necessary adjustments to your anti-inflammatory diet.

3 Cultural and personal preferences: An anti-inflammatory diet can be adapted to fit a variety of cultural and personal food preferences. Focus on incorporating anti-inflammatory principles into your favorite dishes and meal traditions, and don't be afraid to experiment with new recipes and ingredients.

4 Nutrient needs: Depending on your age, gender, and life stage, you may have different nutrient requirements. For example, pregnant and breastfeeding women, older adults, and athletes may have higher needs for certain vitamins, minerals, and macronutrients. Consider working with a registered dietitian to ensure your anti-inflammatory diet is meeting your specific nutrient needs.

5 Lifestyle factors: Your anti-inflammatory diet should fit seamlessly into your lifestyle and take into account factors such as your work schedule, family obligations, and social life. Make adjustments as needed to ensure your diet is realistic and sustainable for you.

Remember, an anti-inflammatory diet is not a one-size-fits-all approach. By customizing your diet to your unique needs and preferences, you can create a way of eating that is both nourishing and enjoyable, increasing your chances of long-term success.

Reintroducing foods and monitoring reactions If you have eliminated certain foods from your diet as part of an anti-inflammatory protocol, you may eventually wish to reintroduce them to assess your tolerance and expand your dietary options. Reintroducing foods systematically and monitoring your body's reactions can help you determine which foods you can safely include in your diet and which ones you may need to continue avoiding.

Here's a step-by-step guide to reintroducing foods:

1 Choose one food at a time: Select a single food that you have

been avoiding and wish to reintroduce. It's important to introduce foods one at a time to accurately assess your body's response.

2 Start with a small amount: Begin by consuming a small portion of the food, such as a teaspoon or tablespoon, depending on the food. This allows you to gauge your body's reaction to the food without overwhelming your system.

3 Monitor your symptoms: Over the next 24-48 hours, pay close attention to any symptoms or reactions you may experience, such as digestive issues, skin irritation, headaches, or joint pain. Keep a food and symptom journal to track your body's response.

4 Gradually increase the amount: If you do not experience any adverse reactions, gradually increase the portion size of the food over the next few days, continuing to monitor your symptoms closely.

5 Decide whether to include or avoid the food: If you are able to consume the food without any negative reactions, you can choose to include it in your anti-inflammatory diet. However, if you experience symptoms or discomfort, it may be best to continue avoiding that food and focus on other nourishing options.

6 Repeat the process: Once you have successfully reintroduced or eliminated one food, move on to the next food you wish to test, following the same systematic approach.

Remember, everyone's body is different, and what works for one person may not work for another. Trust your body's signals and be patient with the reintroduction process. If you have any concerns or experience severe reactions, consult with a healthcare professional for guidance.

Continuous learning and staying informed The field of nutrition and health is constantly evolving, with new research and insights emerging all the time. To maintain long-term success with your anti-inflammatory diet and lifestyle, it's essential to stay informed and continue learning about the latest developments and best practices.

Here are some ways to stay informed and continue expanding your knowledge:

1 Read reputable sources: Seek out reliable, science-based information from trusted sources, such as academic journals, reputable

health organizations, and qualified healthcare professionals. Be cautious of sensationalized media headlines or unsubstantiated claims from unqualified individuals.

2 Attend workshops and seminars: Participate in workshops, seminars, and conferences that focus on anti-inflammatory living, nutrition, and holistic health. These events can provide valuable insights, practical tips, and networking opportunities with like-minded individuals.

3 Follow trusted experts: Follow qualified healthcare professionals, researchers, and thought leaders in the field of integrative and anti-inflammatory medicine on social media, blogs, and podcasts. This can help you stay up-to-date on the latest research, trends, and best practices.

4 Engage with a supportive community: Connect with others who are following an anti-inflammatory lifestyle through online forums, social media groups, or local meetups. Sharing experiences, recipes, and support can enhance your learning and keep you motivated.

5 Experiment and adapt: As you continue to learn and gain insights, be open to experimenting with new foods, recipes, and lifestyle practices that align with anti-inflammatory principles. Adapt your approach as needed based on your body's responses and your evolving knowledge.

6 Work with professionals: Consider partnering with qualified healthcare professionals, such as registered dietitians, functional medicine practitioners, or holistic nutritionists, who can provide personalized guidance and help you stay informed about the latest research and best practices.

By committing to continuous learning and staying informed, you can deepen your understanding of anti-inflammatory living, refine your approach, and maximize the long-term benefits of this healthy lifestyle.

Celebrating your progress and health improvements Adopting an anti-inflammatory diet and lifestyle is a significant accomplishment that deserves to be celebrated. Recognizing your progress and health improvements can help keep you motivated, inspired, and committed to your journey.

Here are some ways to celebrate your success:

1 Reflect on your progress: Take time to regularly reflect on how far you've come since starting your anti-inflammatory journey. Consider the positive changes you've made, the challenges you've overcome, and the health benefits you've experienced.

2 Set milestones and reward yourself: Establish specific milestones along your journey, such as completing a 30-day anti-inflammatory diet challenge or achieving a personal health goal. When you reach these milestones, reward yourself with something meaningful and aligned with your values, such as a massage, a new cookbook, or a nature hike with friends.

3 Share your success with others: Don't be afraid to share your progress and health improvements with your loved ones and support system. Celebrating your success with others can help reinforce your commitment and inspire them to prioritize their own health and well-being.

4 Practice gratitude: Cultivate a sense of gratitude for your body, your health, and the nourishing foods and lifestyle practices that support your well-being. Keep a gratitude journal or take a moment each day to reflect on the positive aspects of your anti-inflammatory journey.

5 Pay it forward: Consider sharing your knowledge and experience with others who may benefit from an anti-inflammatory lifestyle. This can include sharing recipes, offering support and encouragement, or volunteering with local health organizations. Helping others can deepen your own commitment and sense of purpose.

6 Embrace a growth mindset: Remember that your anti-inflammatory journey is an ongoing process of learning, growth, and self-discovery. Embrace challenges and setbacks as opportunities for learning and refinement, and celebrate your resilience and adaptability.

By taking the time to celebrate your progress and health improvements, you can maintain a positive outlook, stay motivated, and continue to thrive on your anti-inflammatory journey.

Conclusion Long-term success with an anti-inflammatory diet and lifestyle requires dedication, customization, continuous learning, and a celebration of progress. By staying committed to your goals, tailoring your approach to your unique needs and preferences, staying informed about the latest research and best practices, and recognizing your achievements, you can create a sustainable and deeply rewarding way of life.

Remember, an anti-inflammatory lifestyle is not about perfection but rather about consistently making choices that nourish your body, mind, and spirit. Embrace the journey, be patient with yourself, and trust in the transformative power of small, daily actions.

As you continue on your anti-inflammatory path, keep in mind that you are not alone. Surround yourself with a supportive community of like-minded individuals who share your values and goals, and don't hesitate to seek guidance from qualified healthcare professionals when needed.

By making your anti-inflammatory diet and lifestyle a long-term priority, you can experience profound improvements in your health, vitality, and overall quality of life. Celebrate your commitment to self-care and wellness, and know that every step you take toward nourishing your body and reducing inflammation is a powerful investment in your future health and happiness.

CONCLUSION

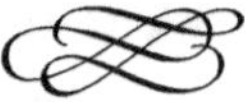

Congratulations on your journey towards adopting an anti-inflammatory lifestyle! By reaching this final chapter, you have demonstrated a strong commitment to improving your health and well-being. You have learned about the science behind inflammation, the foods that contribute to or reduce inflammation, and the lifestyle factors that play a crucial role in managing chronic inflammation. You have also discovered practical strategies for implementing an anti-inflammatory diet, navigating social situations, and tailoring your approach to address specific health concerns.

Now, as you embark on the long-term maintenance of your anti-inflammatory lifestyle, it is essential to focus on the key factors that will ensure your ongoing success. This chapter will provide you with valuable insights and strategies for staying committed, customizing your approach, reintroducing foods, continuing your education, and celebrating your progress. By incorporating these elements into your anti-inflammatory journey, you will be well-equipped to maintain your health improvements and enjoy a vibrant, fulfilling life.

Section 1: Staying Committed to the Anti-Inflammatory Lifestyle Maintaining an anti-inflammatory lifestyle requires dedication, perseverance, and a strong sense of purpose. While you may have experienced significant improvements in your health and well-being during your initial transition, it is common to face challenges and obstacles along the way. To ensure long-term success, it is crucial to develop strategies that will keep you motivated and committed to your goals.

1.1 Setting Clear and Achievable Goals One of the most effective ways to stay committed to your anti-inflammatory lifestyle is to set clear and achievable goals. These goals should be specific, measurable, attainable, relevant, and time-bound (SMART). For example, instead of setting a vague goal like "I want to be healthier," you might set a specific goal such as "I will incorporate at least five servings of anti-inflammatory fruits and vegetables into my diet every day for the next three months."

When setting your goals, consider both short-term and long-term objectives. Short-term goals, such as trying a new anti-inflammatory recipe each week or engaging in 30 minutes of physical activity every day, can help you build momentum and stay motivated. Long-term goals, such as reducing your inflammation markers or achieving remission of an autoimmune condition, can provide a sense of direction and purpose for your anti-inflammatory journey.

Remember to be realistic and compassionate with yourself when setting goals. It is important to challenge yourself, but also to acknowledge that progress may be gradual and that setbacks are a normal part of the process. Celebrate your achievements along the way and use any obstacles as opportunities for learning and growth.

1.2 Building a Strong Support System Having a strong support system is crucial for maintaining an anti-inflammatory lifestyle. Surrounding yourself with people who understand and support your health goals can provide encouragement, accountability, and motivation when you need it most.

Start by sharing your anti-inflammatory journey with your loved ones. Explain why you have chosen to adopt this lifestyle and how it benefits your health and well-being. Invite them to join you in preparing healthy meals, engaging in physical activity, and exploring new ways to manage stress and promote relaxation.

In addition to your immediate family and friends, consider joining a community of like-minded individuals who are also pursuing an anti-inflammatory lifestyle. This can include online forums, social media groups, or local meetups focused on healthy living. Connecting with others who share your values and goals can provide a wealth of support, inspiration, and practical advice.

If you are facing specific health challenges or concerns, consider seeking support from professionals such as registered dietitians, functional medicine practitioners, or health coaches who specialize in anti-inflammatory protocols. These experts can provide personalized guidance, help you navigate challenges, and ensure that you are following an evidence-based approach to managing your health.

1.3 Prioritizing Self-Care and Stress Management Self-care and stress management are essential components of an anti-inflammatory lifestyle. Chronic stress can contribute to inflammation in the body, undermining the benefits of a healthy diet and lifestyle. To stay committed to your anti-inflammatory journey, it is crucial to prioritize activities that promote relaxation, reduce stress, and support overall well-being.

Incorporate stress-reducing practices into your daily routine, such as:

- Mindfulness meditation
- Deep breathing exercises
- Progressive muscle relaxation
- Yoga or tai chi
- Spending time in nature
- Engaging in hobbies or creative pursuits
- Connecting with loved ones
- Practicing gratitude

Make self-care a non-negotiable part of your schedule, just like any other important appointment or commitment. Set aside time each day for activities that nourish your mind, body, and spirit, and be proactive in managing your stress levels.

Remember that self-care also involves setting healthy boundaries, saying no to commitments that don't align with your values or health goals, and asking for help when you need it. By prioritizing your own well-being, you will be better equipped to stay committed to your anti-inflammatory lifestyle and navigate any challenges that arise.

1.4 Planning and Preparation Planning and preparation are key to staying committed to your anti-inflammatory lifestyle, especially when life becomes busy or stressful. By taking the time to plan your meals, stock your kitchen with healthy options, and prepare food in advance, you can ensure that you always have nourishing choices available and reduce the temptation to resort to inflammatory convenience foods.

Set aside time each week to plan your meals and snacks, focusing on incorporating a variety of anti-inflammatory foods such as fruits, vegetables, whole grains, lean proteins, and healthy fats. Use this time to research new recipes, make a grocery list, and identify any prep work that can be done in advance, such as washing and chopping vegetables, cooking whole grains, or preparing homemade sauces or dressings.

Consider batch cooking or meal prepping on weekends or during less busy times, so that you have ready-to-eat options available throughout the week. This can include preparing large batches of soups, stews, or casseroles that can be portioned and frozen for later use, or assembling individual meals or snacks that can be easily grabbed on the go.

Keep your kitchen stocked with anti-inflammatory staples, such as fresh and frozen fruits and vegetables, whole grains, legumes, nuts and seeds, and healthy oils, so that you always have the ingredients on hand to create nourishing meals and snacks.

By dedicating time to planning and preparation, you can reduce stress, save time, and ensure that you are consistently fueling your body with the nutrients it needs to combat inflammation and support optimal health.

Section 2: Customizing the Diet to Your Needs An anti-inflammatory diet is not a one-size-fits-all approach. While the general principles of emphasizing whole, nutrient-dense foods and minimizing processed, inflammatory foods apply to everyone, the specific foods and dietary patterns that work best for you may vary based on your individual needs, preferences, and health status.

2.1 Addressing Food Sensitivities and Allergies Food sensitivities and allergies can contribute to inflammation in the body and exacerbate a range of health conditions. If you suspect that certain foods may be triggering symptoms or undermining your health progress, it is important to work with a healthcare professional to identify and address these sensitivities.

Common food sensitivities that can contribute to inflammation include:

- Gluten (found in wheat, barley, and rye)
- Dairy (particularly cow's milk)
- Soy
- Eggs
- Corn
- Peanuts
- Shellfish

If you have a confirmed food allergy or sensitivity, it is essential to eliminate the offending foods from your diet completely. This may require careful label reading, communication with restaurants or food service providers, and the development of alternative meal and snack options.

If you suspect a food sensitivity but have not yet identified the specific trigger, consider working with a healthcare professional to conduct an elimination diet. This involves removing suspected trigger foods from your diet for a period of time (typically 3-4 weeks) and then systematically reintroducing them one at a time while monitoring for symptoms. This process can help you identify which foods may be contributing to inflammation and other health issues.

2.2 Tailoring Your Diet to Specific Health Conditions Certain health conditions may require specific dietary modifications to optimize the anti-inflammatory benefits of your diet. For example:

- Autoimmune conditions: If you have an autoimmune condition such as rheumatoid arthritis, lupus, or multiple sclerosis, you may benefit from a more targeted anti-inflammatory approach such as the autoimmune protocol (AIP). This protocol eliminates common inflammatory triggers such as grains, legumes, dairy, eggs, nuts, seeds, and nightshade vegetables for a period of time before carefully reintroducing them to assess tolerance.

• Cardiovascular disease: If you have or are at risk for heart disease, you may benefit from a diet that emphasizes heart-healthy fats such as olive oil and fatty fish, fiber-rich foods such as fruits, vegetables, and whole grains, and limits saturated and trans fats, added sugars, and sodium.

• Digestive disorders: If you have a digestive condition such as inflammatory bowel disease (IBD), celiac disease, or irritable bowel syndrome (IBS), you may need to tailor your anti-inflammatory diet to address specific triggers or nutritional needs. This may involve eliminating certain foods, such as gluten or FODMAPs (fermentable oligosaccharides, disaccharides, monosaccharides, and polyols), or incorporating foods that support gut healing, such as bone broth or fermented foods.

• Neurological conditions: If you have a neurological condition such as Alzheimer's disease, Parkinson's disease, or multiple sclerosis, you may benefit from a diet that emphasizes brain-healthy nutrients such as omega-3 fatty acids, antioxidants, and B vitamins. The MIND (Mediterranean-DASH Intervention for Neurodegenerative Delay) diet, which combines elements of the Mediterranean and DASH (Dietary Approaches to Stop Hypertension) diets, has been shown to support brain health and reduce the risk of cognitive decline.

When tailoring your anti-inflammatory diet to address specific health conditions, it is important to work closely with a healthcare professional who can provide personalized guidance and ensure that your nutritional needs are being met. Remember that dietary modifications should be used in conjunction with, not as a replacement for, appropriate medical treatment and monitoring.

2.3 Considering Cultural and Personal Preferences An anti-inflammatory diet can be adapted to a wide range of cultural and personal food preferences. The key is to focus on incorporating anti-inflammatory principles into your existing dietary patterns and favorite dishes, rather than feeling restricted or deprived.

Some strategies for adapting an anti-inflammatory diet to your cultural and personal preferences include:

• Emphasizing traditional, whole-food ingredients: Many traditional cuisines around the world feature anti-inflammatory ingredients such as fresh fruits and vegetables, whole grains, legumes, and healthy fats. Focus on incorporating these whole-food ingredients into your favorite dishes, while minimizing processed or refined elements.

• Experimenting with new flavors and spices: Herbs and spices are rich in anti-inflammatory compounds and can add depth and complexity to your meals. Explore new flavors and spice combinations from different culinary traditions to keep your anti-inflammatory diet interesting and varied.

• Modifying recipes to increase nutrient density: Look for opportunities to boost the anti-inflammatory potential of your favorite recipes by adding or substituting ingredients. For example, you might add extra vegetables to a pasta dish, swap refined grains for whole grains, or replace heavy cream with coconut milk in a curry.

• Finding healthy alternatives for favorite treats: If you have a sweet tooth or enjoy savory snacks, look for anti-inflammatory alternatives that satisfy your cravings without compromising your health goals. This might include dark chocolate, fresh fruit, roasted nuts, or air-popped popcorn.

• Celebrating cultural and social traditions mindfully: Food is often a central part of cultural and social celebrations, and it's important to find ways to participate in these traditions while staying true to your anti-inflammatory goals. Focus on enjoying the company and conversation, and choose the most nourishing options available. If you're attending a potluck or hosting an event, offer to bring an anti-inflammatory dish that everyone can enjoy.

Remember that an anti-inflammatory diet is a flexible, lifelong approach to nourishing your body and promoting optimal health. By finding ways to incorporate anti-inflammatory principles into your existing food culture and preferences, you can create a sustainable, enjoyable way of eating that supports your long-term health and well-being.

Section 3: Reintroducing Foods and Monitoring Reactions As you become more comfortable with your anti-inflammatory diet and experience improvements in your health and well-being, you may wish to reintroduce some of the foods you initially eliminated. This process can help you identify which foods you may be able to tolerate in moderation and which foods are best avoided for optimal health.

3.1 The Reintroduction Process When reintroducing foods, it's important to do so systematically and mindfully, paying close attention to your body's reactions. A typical reintroduction process involves the following steps:

1 Choose one food to reintroduce at a time: Select a food that you have been avoiding as part of your anti-inflammatory diet, such as gluten, dairy, or soy.

2 Start with a small amount: Begin by consuming a small portion of the food, such as a teaspoon or tablespoon, depending on the food.

3 Monitor your reactions: Pay close attention to any symptoms or changes in your body over the next 24-48 hours. These may include digestive symptoms (bloating, gas, diarrhea, constipation), skin reactions (rash, itching, acne), respiratory symptoms (congestion, sneezing, coughing), joint pain or stiffness, headaches, fatigue, or changes in mood or mental clarity.

4 Gradually increase the amount: If you do not experience any adverse reactions, gradually increase the portion size of the food over the next few days, continuing to monitor your body's response.

5 Decide whether to include or avoid the food: If you are able to consume the food without any negative reactions, you may choose to include it in your anti-inflammatory diet in moderation. However, if you experience symptoms or discomfort, it may be best to continue avoiding that food for optimal health.

6 Repeat the process: Once you have successfully reintroduced or eliminated one food, move on to the next food you wish to test, following the same systematic approach.

It's important to note that the reintroduction process can take time and may require patience and persistence. Some reactions may be delayed or subtle, so it's important to pay close attention to your body's signals and be willing to make adjustments as needed.

3.2 Keeping a Food and Symptom Journal Keeping a food and symptom journal can be a valuable tool for monitoring your body's reactions during the reintroduction process and beyond. By tracking the foods you eat and any symptoms or changes you experience, you can identify patterns and make connections between your diet and your health.

To keep a food and symptom journal, follow these steps:

1 Record everything you eat and drink: Write down all the foods and beverages you consume throughout the day, including portion sizes and any relevant details (e.g., brand names, preparation methods).

2 Note any symptoms or changes: Pay attention to any physical, mental, or emotional symptoms you experience, such as digestive issues, skin reactions, energy levels, mood, or sleep quality. Record these symptoms in your journal, along with the time they occurred and any other relevant details.

3 Look for patterns: After several days or weeks of tracking, review your journal to identify any patterns or connections between the foods you eat and the symptoms you experience. For example, you may notice that you consistently experience bloating and gas after consuming dairy products, or that you have more energy and mental clarity on days when you eat more leafy greens.

4 Make adjustments as needed: Based on the patterns you identify, make adjustments to your anti-inflammatory diet as needed. This may involve eliminating certain foods that consistently trigger symptoms or incorporating more of the foods that seem to support your health and well-being.

Remember that a food and symptom journal is a personal tool that can help you tune in to your body's unique needs and responses. Be honest and consistent in your tracking, and be willing to experiment and make changes based on what you learn. If you have any concerns about your symptoms or reactions, don't hesitate to consult with a healthcare professional for guidance and support.

Section 4: Continuous Learning and Staying Informed The field of nutrition and anti-inflammatory living is constantly evolving, with new research and insights emerging all the time. To support your long-term success and maintain your commitment to an anti-inflammatory lifestyle, it's important to stay informed and engage in continuous learning.

4.1 Staying Up-to-Date with Current Research Staying up-to-date with current research can help you make informed decisions about your anti-inflammatory diet and lifestyle, and ensure that you are following evidence-based practices for optimal health. Some strategies for staying informed include:

• Reading reputable health and nutrition publications: Look for articles and studies from respected scientific journals, such as the Journal of Nutrition, the American Journal of Clinical Nutrition, and the Journal of the Academy of Nutrition and Dietetics.

• Following trusted health organizations: Stay informed about the latest recommendations and guidelines from reputable health organizations, such as the World Health Organization (WHO), the National Institutes of Health (NIH), and the Academy of Nutrition and Dietetics.

• Attending conferences and workshops: Participate in conferences, workshops, and webinars that focus on anti-inflammatory nutrition and lifestyle medicine. These events can provide valuable insights and opportunities to learn from leading experts in the field.

• Consulting with healthcare professionals: Work with qualified healthcare professionals, such as registered dietitians, functional medicine practitioners, or integrative medicine physicians, who can provide personalized guidance and keep you informed about the latest research and best practices